Quic

Quick Guide to Transfusion Medicine

Marisa B. Marques, MD
Associate Professor, Department of Pathology
Division of Laboratory Medicine
Transfusion Medicine and Coagulation Services Director
The University of Alabama at Birmingham
Birmingham, Alabama

Margaret G. Fritsma, MA, MT(ASCP)SBB
Associate Professor, Pathology and Clinical Laboratory Sciences
School of Health Professions
Division of Laboratory Medicine
The University of Alabama at Birmingham
Birmingham, Alabama

AACCPress

1850 K Street, NW, Suite 625
Washington, DC 20006

1 2 3 4 5 6 7 8 9 0 EB 09 08 07

Printed in the United States of America

Library of Congress Cataloging-in-Publication Data

Marques, Marisa B.

Quick guide to transfusion medicine/Marisa B. Marques, Margaret G. Fritsma.

p. ; cm.

Includes bibliographical references and index.

ISBN-13: 978-1-59425-073-6

ISBN-10: 1-59425-073-1

1. Blood—Transfusion—Handbooks, manuals, etc. I. Fritsma, Margaret G. II. American Association for Clinical Chemistry. III. Title.

[DNLM: 1. Blood Component Transfusion—methods—Handbooks.

2. Blood Donors—Handbooks. WB 39 M357q 2007]

RM171.M36 2007

615'.39—dc22

2007014206

Preface

The *Quick Guide to Transfusion Medicine* is intended for physicians, nurses, physician assistants, nurse practitioners, medical technologists and pharmacists—and particularly for residents and students in these professions.

As one of the broadest areas of clinical pathology, transfusion medicine includes not only laboratory testing, but also the treatment of a variety of conditions with blood products and blood derivatives. Many individuals who practice transfusion medicine are also involved in donor and/or therapeutic apheresis. We organized the *Guide* to serve as a quick reference to the multiple steps necessary to ensure transfusion safety. It starts with the criteria to select appropriate donors, the preparation of components, testing of the recipient, crossmatching when appropriate, and indications for transfusion in general and in specific patient populations (i.e., neonates) or clinical conditions (i.e., sickle cell anemia), as well as treatment of congenital bleeding disorders (i.e., hemophilia and von Willebrand disease), evaluation and treatment of transfusion reactions, alternatives to patients who refuse transfusion, and therapeutic apheresis. Many references are included to facilitate more in-depth learning of the topics discussed. We hope the readers will find it very useful in daily practice.

Marisa B. Marques
Margaret G. Fritsma

Contents

Transfusion Safety

Introduction

Safe blood transfusion encompasses the whole spectrum of activities, from the collection of blood from the donor, to the final transfusion to the recipient (Table 1). A weakness or breakdown in any step compromises the entire process, and may result in injury to the patient or even death. It is essential that all aspects of blood collection and transfusion are conducted accurately and thoroughly.

Table 1. Multiple steps essential to ensure transfusion safety (1,2)

	Donor Blood Collection
Donor screening	Accurate medical history and physical exam; donor qualification
Blood collection	Correct identification; proper aseptic technique
Donor blood processing	Accurate testing and labeling
Component preparation	Proper methods, labeling, storage, and quality assessment
	Pretransfusion Recipient Testing
Sample collection	Correct patient; proper technique
Sample identification	Two unique patient identifiers; date and time of collection

(Continued)

Table 1. (Continued)

Pretransfusion Recipient Testing (Continued)	
Laboratory testing	Accurate and timely ABO and Rh typing, antibody screen, crossmatch
Ordering physicians	Transfusion trigger; appropriate product/dose/timing
Issuing of Blood	
Nurses	Correctly request what was ordered
Transfusion service	Prepare product appropriately (i.e., irradiation, leukoreduction)
Delivery of product	Release correct product directly to transfusionist
Blood Administration	
Informed consent	Requested prior to placing transfusion order; documented in chart
Venous access	Ready to use; no concurrent medications
Bedside patient identification	Compare patient and blood product information—at least two people: Patient armband identification *vs.* donor unit label *vs.* compatibility label
Patient monitoring	Vital signs before, during, and after transfusion; signs and symptoms of reaction
Posttransfusion	
Follow-up: recognition of late complications	Delayed transfusion reactions; graft-vs.-host disease; infections

There is strong evidence from hemovigilance programs and error-reporting systems that most serious hazards of transfusion result from errors that occur outside the laboratory (3). Nevertheless, studies have shown that almost one-third of errors occur within the transfusion service (4–6) . Examples of these errors are shown in Table 2.

Table 2. Transfusion service errors

Not checking previous records of patients before blood is released
Using the wrong patient sample for testing
Taking shortcuts in procedures or processes (example: perform direct ABO type but omit reverse type)
Making clerical or transcription errors
Placing blood in the wrong location in the refrigerator
Issuing the wrong blood for transfusion
Mixing up patient samples with similar or same last names

Transfusion Safety Officer (TSO)

- Common in France, England, and Canada
- Rare in the United States, although needed
- Ideally, a hospital has two TSOs:
  - One individual (often a technologist) to function as compliance officer
  - A nurse to work outside the transfusion service (blood bank) as a patient safety advocate

Goals and activities of a TSO (1)

- To work interdepartmentally and outside the laboratory to promote safe and effective transfusion therapy
- To track hospital performance of key processes by
  - Active surveillance (observation audits) of patient sample collection, blood requests, blood delivery, and bedside administration of blood components
  - Collection of data on indicators of the transfusion process
  - Participation in organization-wide program of error reporting to the hospital Transfusion Practice Committee and hospital management

- To educate staff (nursing, physician) to recognize and report transfusion reactions and disseminate information on hospital guidelines for appropriate blood usage
- To provide "basic training" for new physician staff responsible for administering blood in high usage areas (e.g., anesthesiology residents, emergency room personnel)
- To contribute to improving processes for blood utilization review
- To participate in implementation of new technology designed to enhance patient safety

Blood Donation, Collection, and Processing

Donor Qualification

On the day of donation, each donor receives a limited physical examination consisting of blood pressure, pulse, temperature, and hemoglobin or hematocrit measurement. Questions are asked regarding the donor's health, medical history, and activities. Guidelines for evaluation of donor eligibility are found in Tables 3 through 8.

Table 3. Criteria for allogeneic blood donation (7–10)

Condition	*Deferral; Comment*
Age	At least 17 years of age; accept 16 years of age if allowed by state law
Allergy	Defer temporarily if breathing difficulty is present
Asthma	Accept if no difficulty breathing and no limitations/restrictions in normal daily activities
Blood pressure	Systolic: ≤180 mm Hg; diastolic: ≤100 mm Hg
Pulse	50–100 beats/minute; no irregularity. <50 bpm in healthy athlete
Temperature	≤37.5 °C (99.5 °F)
Hemoglobin/hematocrit	≥12.5 g/dL / ≥38%
Heart, liver, lung, or other organ disease; cancer; abnormal bleeding tendency	Defer, unless determined suitable by medical director

(Continued)

Table 3. (Continued)

Condition	*Deferral; Comment*
Donation interval	8 weeks after whole blood donation 16 weeks after double red cell collection 4 weeks after infrequent plasmapheresis >2 days after plasmapheresis, plateletpheresis, or leukapheresis
Dental work	Accept teeth cleaning, scaling, root canal, fillings, and tooth extraction, if no infection present Defer 3 days for oral surgery, abscesses, or infection
Diabetes	Use of insulin pump may be acceptable Defer indefinitely if, since 1980, received an injection of bovine (beef) insulin made from cattle from Europe
Heart/lung disease	Defer for 1 year after the last symptom of sarcoidosis Defer for 6 months from last symptom/medical evaluation/restrictions on activities for most heart disease such as murmur, angina, valvular insufficiency, coronary artery bypass surgery, arrhythmia, aneurysm, cardiac catheterization, congestive heart failure, heart attack, stroke, transient ischemic attack, pacemaker Defer temporarily if symptomatic or has restrictions on activities for most lung diseases
Infectious diseases	See Tables 4 and 5
Immunizations	See Table 6
Medications	See Table 7

Condition	*Deferral; Comment*
Pregnancy	Defer while pregnant Defer for 6 weeks after uncomplicated third trimester term delivery or cesarean section Defer for 12 months if delivery required a blood transfusion Accept nursing mothers
Sickle cell disease	Defer for sickle cell disease Accept for sickle cell trait
Skin disease and rash	Donors will be individually evaluated Phlebotomy site must be free of rash/skin disease
Surgery	Accept history of recent surgery if: • Underlying illness does not disqualify donor • Stitches/staples dissolved or removed • Donor has resumed normal activity and is feeling well • Donor did not receive a blood transfusion or transplant Accept minor cuts requiring stitches/staples after 48 hours, if no signs of infection
Tattoo/pocketing/body piercing	Tattoo is acceptable if: • Applied in a state that regulates tattoo facilities AND • Donor states the tattoo was applied by a regulated facility AND • Applied with sterile, single-use needles and ink, OR • If more than 12 months since procedure

(Continued)

Table 3. (Continued)

Condition	*Deferral; Comment*
	Pocketing is acceptable if: • Needles, teflon, and instruments used were all sterile OR • If more than 12 months since procedure Ear/body piercing (including acupuncture and electrolysis) is acceptable if: • Sterile, single-use needles were used OR • More than 12 months since the procedure
Transfusion/transplant/ needle-stick	Defer 12 months Receipt of human dura mater—defer indefinitely
Travel	See Table 8
Weight/height	Minimum 110 lbs. for whole blood donation Maximum of 10.5 mL of blood collected/kg of donor weight Minimum for double red cell donation: • Males: at least 150 lbs. and 5'1" in height • Females: at least 175 lbs. and 5'5" in height Maximum acceptable weight on most donation chairs is 350 lbs. Few locations have chairs suitable to accommodate donors larger than 350 lbs.

Table 4. Deferral criteria to prevent HIV transmission (7–10)

Any person who has had sex with any person with HIV or at high risk of HIV From date of release from lock-up, jail, prison, or juvenile detention center (including work release) if held more than 72 consecutive hours Mucous membrane or skin penetration exposure to another person's blood	Defer 12 months
Any person who has ever had a positive test for HIV Any person who has AIDS or one of its symptoms, which include: • Unexplained weight loss (10 pounds or more in less than 2 months) • Night sweats • Blue or purple spots on or under the skin or in the mouth • Long-lasting white spots or unusual mouth sores • Lumps in the neck, armpits, or groin that lasted more than a month • Fever higher than 100.5 °F (38.05 °C) that lasted more than 10 days • Diarrhea lasting over a month • Persistent cough and shortness of breath Any person who has used needles, even once, to take drugs, steroids, or anything not prescribed by a doctor Male who has ever had sex, even once, with another male since 1977 Any person who has been given money, drugs, or other payment for sex since 1977	Defer indefinitely

(Continued)

Table 4. (Continued)

Any person who was born in or lived in Cameroon, Central African Republic, Chad, Congo, Equatorial Guinea, Gabon, Niger, or Nigeria since 1977 for 5 years or more
Any person who received blood transfusions in any of the above countries since 1977
Any person who had sex with anyone who was born in or lived in any of the above countries
Any person who had clotting factor concentrates for therapy of a bleeding disorder such as hemophilia

Table 5. Deferral criteria to prevent transmission of infections other than HIV (7–10)

Infection	*Deferral; Comment*
Cold, flu, or sore throat	Defer temporarily for active cold or flu symptoms such as fever, sore throat, productive cough, or general fatigue on day of donation
Creutzfeldt-Jakob disease (CJD)	Defer indefinitely if at increased risk for, a history of, a diagnosis of, or have any blood relatives diagnosed with CJD See Table 8 (Travel outside the U.S.)
Hepatitis	Defer indefinitely for viral hepatitis after 11th birthday Accept if: • Jaundice or hepatitis associated with birth, medications, or bile duct obstruction • Hepatitis of unknown type before 11th birthday

Infection	*Deferral; Comment*
Exposure to hepatitis/ HIV/AIDS	Defer 12 months: • From last contact with another person's blood into open wound and/or non intact skin and/or mucous membrane (this includes sharing razors or toothbrushes and occupational exposure) • Following human bite or primate (ape family) animal bite that broke the skin • Accidental exposure to needle/instrument contaminated with blood from another person/primate • From last sexual contact with anyone diagnosed with HIV/AIDS, hepatitis, or who is a hepatitis B carrier • From last contact if lived with (resided in same house, apartment, dormitory, etc.) person with hepatitis or is chronic hepatitis B carrier • From date of release from lock-up, jail, prison, or juvenile detention center (including work release) if held more than 72 consecutive hours
Malaria	Defer 12 months after travel to endemic area Defer 3 years after living 5 consecutive years in country endemic for malaria Defer 3 years after symptom/treatment
Syphilis	Defer 12 months after positive test and treatment
West Nile virus	Refer to FDA Guidance
Babesiosis	Defer indefinitely
Chagas disease	Defer indefinitely

Table 6. Deferral criteria based on history of immunizations (7–10)

Toxoids, synthetic or killed vaccines (anthrax, cholera, diphtheria, HAV, HBV, influenza, Lyme disease, paratyphoid, pertussis, plague, pneumococcal, polio, Rocky Mountain Spotted Fever, tetanus, typhoid)	No deferral, if symptom-free and afebrile
Red measles (rubeola) Mumps Oral polio Typhoid Yellow fever	Defer for 2 weeks
German measles (rubella) MMR (measles, mumps, and rubella) Varivax (chicken pox)	Defer for 4 weeks
Smallpox	Defer for 8 weeks after vaccination or close contact with vaccination site of anyone else and symptoms developed. Refer to FDA guidance

Table 7. Deferral criteria according to medications (10,11)

Aspirin Other anti-platelet medication	Platelet apheresis donors must wait 36 hours after taking aspirin or aspirin products. Other anti-platelet medication deferral as defined by medical director
Antibiotics (oral or intramuscular)	No deferral if course of medication is completed and donor is asymptomatic
Prophylactic antibiotics	No deferral
Antifungals	No deferral if course of medication is completed and donor is asymptomatic
Antivirals	No deferral if course of medication is completed and donor is asymptomatic
Anticoagulants	Defer for 7 days since last dose
Accutane, Amnesteen, Claravis, Sotret (isotretinoin)	Defer for 1 month
Proscar, Propecia (finasteride)	Defer for 1 month
Avodart (dutasteride)	Defer for 6 months from last dose
Hepatitis B immune globulin	Defer 12 months
Unlicensed vaccine	Defer 1 year or refer to medical director
Soriatane (acitretin)	Defer for 3 years from last dose
Pituitary-derived human growth hormone	Defer indefinitely
Tegison (etretinate)	Defer indefinitely
Pituitary-derived thyrotropin	Defer indefinitely
Bovine insulin	Defer indefinitely

Table 8. Criteria to defer donors based on travel outside the United States (7–10)

Area of Travel	*Deferral*
Travel into an area endemic for malaria	Defer for 12 months
Travel or residency in Iraq due to possible Leishmaniasis exposure	
Previous residency in any country endemic for malaria	Defer for 3 years, if no symptoms of malaria
Cumulative time spent (visited or lived) of 3 months or more in the United Kingdom (UK) from January 1, 1980, through December 31, 1996	Defer indefinitely
Former or current members of the U.S. Military, civilian military employee, or dependent of a member of the U.S. Military who spent a total time of 6 months or more on or associated with a military base in: • Germany, Belgium, and the Netherlands (Holland) from 1980 through 1990 • Greece, Turkey, Spain, Portugal, and Italy from 1980 through 1996	
Cumulative time spent (visited or lived) of 5 years or more in Europe (UK from 1980 through 1996) from January 1, 1980, to the present	
Born in, traveled to, or lived in these African countries after 1977: Cameroon, Central African Republic, Chad, Congo, Equatorial Guinea, Gabon, Niger, or Nigeria	
Received blood or medical treatment involving blood in the African countries listed above	
Received blood in the UK or France from 1980 to present	

Allogeneic Donation

Allogeneic donation is the collection of blood from qualified donors for component preparation, storage, distribution, and patient transfusion. Approximately 450–500 mL of blood is collected into 63–70 mL of CPDA-1 anticoagulant (Table 9). Allogeneic donors are the backbone of the nation's blood supply. An estimated eight million volunteer donors give more than 15 million units of blood annually in the U.S. (12). See Tables 3 through 8 for eligibility criteria and Tables 10 and 11 for testing requirements for allogeneic donation.

Table 9. Composition of solutions used in blood collection and RBC preparation

	*Anticoagulant-Preservative Solutions (mg/63 mL)**			*Content of Additive Solutions (mg/100 mL)***		
	CPD	*CP2D*	*CPDA-1*	*AS-1 (Adsol)*	*AS-3 (Nutricel)*	*AS-5 (Optisol)*
FDA-approved shelf life (days)	21	21	35	42	42	42
Sodium citrate	1,660	1,660	1,660	0	588	0
Citric acid	206	206	206	0	42	0
Dextrose	1,610	3,220	2,010	2,200	1,100	900
Monobasic sodium phosphate	140	140	140	0	276	0
Adenine	0	0	17.3	27	30	30
Mannitol	0	0	0	750	0	525
Sodium chloride	0	0	0	900	410	877

*Added to 450 mL whole blood at time of collection

**Added to RBCs after processing from whole blood

Allogeneic Donor Blood Processing

Each donation must be tested for ABO and Rh type, unexpected blood group antibodies (Table 10), and transfusion-transmissible diseases (Table 11).

Table 10. Serologic testing requirements (8)

ABO type	Test for red cell antigens with anti-A and anti-B reagents
	Test for expected antibodies in serum or plasma with A1 and B reagent red cells
Rh type	Test for D antigen with anti-D reagent
	If anti-D test is negative, test for weak D
	Unit is labeled Rh Positive if either test is positive
Antibody screen	Use methods that demonstrate clinically significant antibodies, and appropriate controls

Table 11. Infectious disease tests (7,8)

Infection	*Test*
Hepatitis C (HCV)	Nucleic acid testing (NAT) for HCV RNA
	Antibody to hepatitis C virus (anti-HCV)
Hepatitis B (HBV)	Hepatitis B surface antigen (HBsAg)
	Antibody to hepatitis B core antigen (Anti-HBc)
HIV	NAT for HIV-1 RNA
	Antibodies to HIV-1 and HIV-2
HTLV I/II	Antibodies to HTLV-I/II
Syphilis	Treponemal and cardiolipin antibodies
West Nile virus	NAT for WNV RNA
Trypanosoma cruzi (Chagas disease)	Antibody to T. cruzi
Cytomegalovirus (CMV)	Antibody to CMV (supplemental test)

Autologous Donation

Autologous donation is the collection and use of the recipient's own blood for his/her transfusion needs. Autologous donation prevents sensitization to foreign red cell or white cell antigens (alloimmunization), transmission of infectious disease, and some adverse transfusion reactions. However, it does not eliminate the risks of bacterial contamination or of misidentification of the blood. Autologous donation can be *preoperative*, in which units of blood are collected and stored prior to elective surgery, or *perioperative*, in which blood is collected and reinfused during surgery (intraoperative) or following surgery (postoperative). See Table 12 for requirements related to preoperative autologous donation.

Table 12. Eligibility, testing, and labeling requirements for autologous donation (8)

Physician order	Required
Hemoglobin and hematocrit	Minimum 11 g/dL and 33%
Pregnancy	Not a contraindication
Frequency	For preoperative, donations must be completed more than 72 hours before the anticipated surgery
Condition with risk of bacteremia	Defer
Testing:	
• ABO and Rh	• Performed by the collecting facility and confirmed by the transfusing facility, if different
• Infectious diseases	• Tests for HBsAg, anti-HBc, anti-HCV, HCV RNA, anti-HIV-1/2, HIV-1 RNA, anti-HTLV-I/II, and syphilis must be performed on at least the first unit collected during a 30-day period, if the unit will be transfused outside the collecting facility

(Continued)

Table 12. (Continued)

Labeling	"Autologous Donor," on tie-tag or label "For Autologous Use Only," if unit is not suitable for allogeneic use "Biohazard," for confirmed positive or repeatedly reactive infectious disease tests "Donor Untested," if infectious disease testing has not been performed "Donor Tested within the Last 30 Days," when the unit has not been tested but the donor has been tested within 30 days of collection

Directed Donation

Directed donation is the collection of blood from an individual for use by a designated recipient within a specified time. Directed donors must meet all the testing and eligibility requirements for allogeneic donation. If the directed donation is not used by the designated recipient, the blood is released for allogeneic use. Directed donations from blood relatives must be irradiated to prevent transfusion-associated graft vs. host disease.

Blood Components

Red Blood Cells (RBCs)

Description

- RBCs prepared from one unit of whole blood donation with 225–250 mL of plasma removed
- Standard unit volume: 250–330 mL
- Stored in anticoagulant-preservative (CPDA-1) and additive solutions (AS) to maintain viability
- RBCs in CPDA-1 contain about 200 mL of red blood cells in 50–70 mL of plasma and anticoagulant-preservative, with a hematocrit of ≤80%. Shelf-life is 35 days at 1–6 °C
- RBCs in AS contain about 200 mL of red blood cells in 100 mL of additive solution, with a hematocrit of ~60%. Shelf-life is 42 days at 1–6 °C
- Expected effect in non-bleeding adult: 1 g/dL hemoglobin or 3% hematocrit increase per unit
- Changes during storage
    - Reduced deformability
    - Increased fragility
    - Shortened life span
    - Release of antioxidant
    - Depleted 2,3-diphosphoglycerate levels and ATP
    - Low p50 that increases affinity of hemoglobin for oxygen and thereby reduces oxygen release to tissues

Indications

- Acute bleeding with blood loss of ≥15% of blood volume with/without a pulse >100 bpm or decrease in systolic BP ≥20%
- Chronic symptomatic anemia
- Anemia prior to anesthesia or elective surgery

Leukocyte-Reduced Blood Products

Description

RBCs or platelets processed to contain $<5 \times 10^6$ residual leukocytes. Other names: leukoreduced, leukofiltered, "CMV safe."
Methods of leukoreduction:

- Prestorage leukoreduction with specific filters, 99.99% efficient, performed at 4 °C in the blood center
- Bedside leukofiltration, 99.9% leukocyte removal
- Washing, 90–99% removal
- Glycerolizing/deglycerolizing, same as washing

Indications

- To decrease chance of febrile non-hemolytic transfusion reactions
- To prevent CMV transmission, considered CMV-safe
- To reduce risk of HLA alloimmunization, important for patients who may require long-term platelet transfusion support and/or solid organ transplants

CMV-Negative Blood Products

Description

RBCs or platelets from donors who test negative for antibodies to CMV. Difficult to procure because majority of donors have been exposed to CMV and will have IgG anti-CMV.

Indications

Should be reserved for patients with the highest risk of contracting CMV infection such as the following:

- Intrauterine transfusions
- Neonatal exchange transfusions
- Infants 0–4 months old
- Allogeneic bone marrow transplant patients when the recipient is CMV negative
- Liver transplant patients <18 years old
- Lung transplant recipients
- Heart-lung transplant recipients
- Heart transplant recipients who are CMV negative
- Cardiovascular surgery patients <12 months old
- Upon request, for CMV-negative immunocompromised patients

Irradiated Blood Products

Description

RBCs, platelets, or granulocytes exposed to 2500 cGy gamma irradiation to prevent leukocyte replication and engraftment in patients at risk for transfusion-associated graft vs. host disease (TA-GVHD). Irradiation takes approximately three minutes and should be done when issuing the blood component. If not used immediately, RBCs expire in 28 days from the date of irradiation, or the original expiration date if earlier. Irradiated RBCs suffer damage of the sodium-potassium pump and leak potassium during storage. Depending on how long it has been since irradiation and the patient's serum potassium level, units may be washed before transfusion.

Indications

The following are the most commonly accepted diseases or situations where irradiated blood products are indicated. However, not every transfusion service will irradiate for all of them, for there is not enough evidence in some cases to confirm that they present a high risk for TA-GVHD.

- Congenital cellular immunodeficiency disorders such as DiGeorge's Syndrome
- Neonates from families with previous child known or suspected of having inherited immunodeficiency
- Autologous and allogeneic hematopoietic progenitor cell transplants
- Hodgkin lymphoma
- Granulocyte transfusions
- Intrauterine transfusions
- Postnatal transfusions up to four months after intrauterine transfusions
- Recipients of directed donations from family members
- Low birth weight neonates <1200 grams
- Hematologic malignancies
- HLA-matched or crossmatch-compatible platelet donations
- Current or past exposure to fludarabine, nelarabine, or clofarabine
- Extracorporeal membrane oxygenation (ECMO) treatment

TA-GVHD

- Serious complication of transfusion: mostly fatal due to bone marrow failure and overwhelming infection within 3 weeks
- Symptoms typically start 2–50 days after transfusion
- See Table 32: Delayed complications of transfusion

Red Blood Cells, Washed

Description

- RBCs washed three times and resuspended in saline with a HCT of 70–80%

- Contain <2% of original plasma proteins and approximately 80% of the red cells
- Washed RBCs must be transfused within 24 hours, since they are prepared in an "open system" with risk of bacterial contamination.

Indications

- Neonatal or intrauterine transfusion of irradiated products when more than five hours have elapsed between irradiation and transfusion. Washing removes extracellular potassium to prevent hyperkalemia. Potassium reference range for newborns is 3.5–5.0 mol/L. Beware that heel stick samples may have elevated potassium due to hemolysis.
- Patients with IgA deficiency, if RBCs from an IgA-deficient donor are not available—must wash six times
- Patients with plasma allergy or severe allergic response not controllable with antihistamines—must wash six times

Red Blood Cells, Deglycerolized

Description

- Methodology capable of preserving RBCs for up to 10 years by glycerolization and freezing
- Preferably fresh RBCs (<6 days) are exposed to glycerol at room temperature to allow it to enter the cytoplasm.
- Glycerol prevents formation of intracellular ice crystals and protects the cell from membrane damage and hemolysis.
- Final concentration of glycerol usually 40% w/v
- Can be stored at ≤ −65 °C for up to 10 years
- Thawed in a 37 °C water bath for about 10 minutes, followed by multiple washes with serially decreasing concentrations of hypertonic solution to remove all the glycerol

- After thawing and deglycerolization, shelf-life is 24 hours
- If not used, the unit can potentially be refrozen, depending on its rarity.

Indications

- For patients with antibodies who require rare red cell types, i.e., negative for high-incidence or multiple antigens
  - For example, an O positive patient with hemoglobin SS disease who has had multiple transfusions and has produced anti-C and anti-e:
    Consider that:
      C-negative phenotype: 30% of the donor population
      e-negative phenotype: 2% of the donor population
  - Thus, the chance of finding an O positive, C-negative, e-negative donor is: $0.3 \times 0.02 = 0.006$ or 0.6%.
  - Such units are rarely available from the "liquid" inventory, even of a large transfusion center or blood bank. The most likely source for them is the frozen stock of rare units.
  - For patients with antibodies to high-frequency antigens or multiple antibodies, it is crucial to explain to their physicians how these antibodies impact the ability to find crossmatch-compatible units.
- For neonates receiving transfusion of maternal RBCs due to hemolytic disease of the fetus and newborn caused by an antibody to a high-frequency antigen (e.g. anti-U or anti-k)
- For prolonged storage of autologous units of people with rare blood types, or who will not accept allogeneic RBCs
- Because deglycerolized RBCs are extensively washed, they may be useful for patients with IgA deficiency, paroxysmal nocturnal hemoglobinuria, or patients with a history of allergies to plasma proteins.

Plasma Products: Fresh Frozen Plasma (FFP), 24-Hour Plasma (FP24), Cryo-Poor Plasma (CPP), or Thawed Plasma

Description

FFP and FP24 contain all the coagulation factors and control proteins found in normal plasma in similar composition (13,14). Table 13 compares levels of the labile coagulation factors V and VIII after preparation of FFP and FP24, before freezing.

- FFP and FP24 are prepared by centrifugation and removal of plasma from whole blood donation
  - FFP frozen within 8 hours of collection
  - FP24 frozen within 24 hours of collection
- Both stored at –18 °C for up to 12 months
- Both thawed at 37 °C and stored at 1–6 °C for up to 24 hours
- If not used within 24 hours, labeled as "Thawed Plasma" and used for up to 5 days (Figure 1)
- Volume: range of 200–300 mL
- Must be ABO compatible (Table 23)
- CPP is plasma remaining after removal of cryoprecipitate
- CPP composition: same as FFP or FP24, except for minimal concentration of fibrinogen, factor VIII, von Willebrand factor (VWF), factor XIII, and fibronectin

Table 13. Median levels of factors V and VIII in FFP and FP24 (14)

	FFP	*FP24*
V	94%	80%
VIII	100%	77%

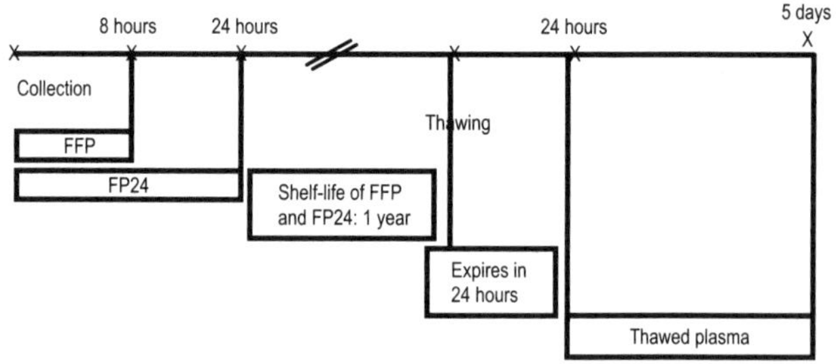

Figure 1. Diagram comparing FFP, FP24, and thawed plasma.

Indications for plasma products

- FFP and FP24 contain all procoagulant and control proteins, including the labile factors V and VIII, and are used for replacement of these proteins in the following coagulopathies. Thawed plasma contains adequate levels of all proteins except factor VIII, and can be used for the same indications (15).
  - Massive transfusion (replacement of ≥1 blood volume within 24 hours)
  - Bleeding in disseminated intravascular coagulation (DIC) with prolonged prothrombin time (PT) and partial thromboplastin time (PTT)
  - Multiple factor deficiencies such as acute or chronic liver failure
  - Bleeding due to warfarin overdose
  - Plasma exchange for thrombotic microangiopathies such as thrombotic thrombocytopenic purpura/hemolytic uremic syndrome (TTP/HUS)
  - Clotting factor deficiencies when factor concentrates are not available
- Adult dose: 10–20 mL/kg body weight (a standard dose would be 4–6 units in an adult). Expect increase of coagulation factor levels by 20%

- Neonates and children dose: 10–15 mL/Kg body weight
- CPP is only used as replacement fluid during plasma exchange for thrombotic thrombocytopenic purpura/hemolytic uremic syndrome (TTP/HUS)

Cryoprecipitate

Description

- Fraction of plasma proteins that precipitate when FFP is thawed in the cold (4 °C)
- Composition: 80–120 units of FVIII, 50% of vWF, and 25% of FXIII from original unit, >150 mg of fibrinogen, and fibronectin (plus residual anti-A and anti-B)
- Volume: 10–15 mL
- Thawed at 37 °C
- Stored at room temperature for up to 6 hours after thawing
- If pooled, transfused within 4 hours
- Preferably ABO-compatible with patient
- Adult dose: 10–20 units; 1 unit/10 kg will increase fibrinogen by 7–10 mg/dL

Indications

- Hypofibrinogenemia, FXIII deficiency, and hypofibronectinemia (burn and traumatic shock patients)
- Von Willebrand disease and hemophilia A should be treated with the corresponding factor concentrates, which have the added safety feature of undergoing viral inactivation steps (see Table 17).
- How to calculate the dose of cryoprecipitate to raise fibrinogen:
  Weight (kg) × 70 mL/kg = blood volume (BV) (mL)
  BV (mL) × (1 − HCT) = plasma volume (PV)(mL)/100 = (dL)
  Mg of fibrinogen required = (desired level in mg/dL − initial level in mg/dL) × PV(dL)
  # units of cryo = mg fibrinogen required/250 mg per unit of cryo

Platelets: Pheresis (Single Donor), Whole Blood-Derived (Random Donor)

Apheresis platelets

- Contents: $\geq 3 \times 10^{11}$ platelets; $<5 \times 10^{6}$ WBC when prestorage leukoreduced; 150 mg fibrinogen in approximately 250 mL of plasma to maintain pH >6.2. Minimal RBC contamination (<0.1 mL)
- Dose: 1 unit/adult or 10–15 mL/kg for neonates
- Expected platelet count increase: Posttransfusion platelet count increase of 30,000/μL. Corrected count increment (CCI) at least 7,500/μL (more likely, 30,000/μL) in 1 hour

Bacterial detection system (BDS): Since March 1, 2004, all apheresis platelet units must be tested on the second day after collection for the presence of contaminating bacteria. Although it is not required that the result be known prior to transfusion, some facilities prefer to wait on transfusion until the initial reading of the culture is shown to be negative. In times of severe shortage, units with pending results may be used after discussing the risks with the patient's physician. If the risk of withholding the transfusion is greater than the historical risk of 1 in 5,000 units being contaminated, the physician should sign that he/she understands the risks and benefits and decides to transfuse the unit. Hospital Transfusion Services may have a specific form that can be called "Emergency Release of Platelet Component, Pending Bacterial Detection Testing" for use in such situations. An example of a statement for the patient's physician to sign follows:

> "I understand the risks involved with transfusion of this platelet component. I feel that the clinical condition of this patient warrants emergency administration of a unit of platelets with pending bacterial detection testing despite the risk involved, and accept full responsibility for the patient outcome."

As soon as the BDS result is available, the transfusion service should notify the patient's physician. In the rare event of a positive test, the patient should be monitored for the possibility of bacteremia.

Random donor platelets (whole blood-derived platelets)

- Contents: ≥5.5 × 10^{10} platelets; <5 × 10^6 WBC (if prestorage leukoreduced); 150 mg fibrinogen in 50–70 mL of plasma to maintain pH >6.2
- Dose: 1 unit/10 kg of body weight for adults and children
- Expected platelet count increase: each unit expected to raise platelet count by 5,000/μL; a pool of 6 units (usual adult dose), expected to achieve an increment of 30,000/μL immediately following the transfusion. CCI at least 7,500/μL in 1 hour

Storage of platelet products

- 5 days at 20–24 °C with agitation
- Chilling of platelets to 4 °C changes membrane conformation and mediates rapid clearance from the circulation through phagocytosis by the reticuloendothelial system. Platelet units placed inadvertently in the refrigerator must be discarded.
- Platelet bags are made of two different materials. The dull side of the bag is the breathable plastic, which allows the platelets to survive storage.
- Each manufactured bag holds a maximum number of platelets to maintain viability. If collection exceeds the limit, one unit must be split and shipped in two connected bags.
- The release of multiple units of apheresis platelets from the transfusion service is discouraged to prevent improper storage of the unit(s) waiting to be transfused.
  - Allow issuing of multiple units in specific clinical situations after discussing with the patient's physician.
  - If possible, check platelet count between units.
- Preparation and storage cause platelet lesion: partial activation and loss of metabolic function

- The longer the storage, the shorter the survival in animals.
- In humans, clinical status of the patient is a more important determinant of recovery and survival.
- Average posttransfusion survival (stored platelets): 6 days

Indications for platelets

- Bleeding due to thrombocytopenia or platelet dysfunction
- Bleeding prophylaxis if platelet count $<10,000/\mu L$ due to bone marrow failure (i.e., associated with leukemia or chemotherapy) or caused by non-immune consumption such as in DIC
- Not recommended in TTP/HUS or heparin-induced thrombocytopenia

Selection of platelets

- First choice: ABO identical. If not available, see Table 14 for best alternatives.
- Due to short shelf-life, inventory is usually more limited than that of RBCs.
- Platelet products contain plasma: transfusion of non-group specific platelets can cause hemolysis due to anti-A and/or anti-B.
- Titer of anti-A and anti-B can be determined by testing 1:50 dilution of unit plasma in saline with A_1 or B cells.
- If no agglutination at 1:50, unit is labeled as "low titer"; can be transfused to patient with corresponding antigen(s)
- If >3 units of ABO mismatched low-titer platelets transfused within 24 hours, increased risk of hemolysis; check DAT (direct antiglobulin test). If positive, perform elution to confirm anti-A and/or anti-B, and evaluate for signs of hemolysis.

Table 14. Choice of platelets based on ABO blood group

Patient Blood Group	*Donor Platelets Blood Group*			
	1st	*2nd*	*3rd*	*Last*
A	A	AB	B	O
B	B	AB	A	O
AB	AB	A	B	O
O	O	AB	A	B

Transfusion of Rh-positive platelets to Rh-negative patients

- Platelets do not have Rh antigens; it is the small number of contaminating RBCs per unit that can sensitize the recipient to form anti-D. Thus, exposure to the D antigen should be avoided in all Rh-negative women of childbearing age.
- If no Rh-negative platelets are available, one vial of Rh immunoglobulin (300 μg) prevents sensitization from as many as 3–5 apheresis units of Rh-positive platelets during a period of 72 hours.
- If intramuscular injection of Rh immunoglobulin is indicated, it should wait until platelet count increases (posttransfusion) to prevent hematoma formation.
- Several recent publications demonstrate that patients with hematologic malignancies and recipients of stem cell transplants do not produce anti-D following transfusion of Rh-positive platelets (16,17).

Platelet refractoriness

Failure to achieve platelet corrected count increment (CCI) of at least 7,500/μL after one unit of apheresis platelets or a dose of random donor platelets. Calculate true platelet response with following formula:

Corrected count increment (CCI) = (platelet count 1 hour posttransfusion – platelet count pretransfusion) × BSA(m^2) / number of platelets × 10^{11} in unit

- Minimum number of 3×10^{11} platelets per apheresis unit. For more accurate number, contact the blood center
- Low CCI at 1 hour suggests antibody-mediated loss
- Platelet loss due to bleeding, fever, or splenomegaly does not usually affect the 1-hour response to a platelet transfusion as antibodies do.
- HLA-matched and crossmatched units are very costly and not readily available. Patient monitoring is required to assess response to transfusion.
- HLA-matching requires donor type; may take several days
- Platelet crossmatching: solid-phase assay based on hemagglutination

Table 15. Causes of immune platelet refractoriness

Type of Antibody	*Associations*	*Laboratory Evaluation*	*Treatment Options*
Alloantibody(ies)	Previous pregnancy and/or transfusion	Indirect platelet antibodies (in serum) followed by antibody specificity test (ELISA)	HLA-matched or crossmatched platelets
Autoantibody	Autoimmune disorder or idiopathic		Intravenous immunoglobulin
Antibody to platelet factor 4-heparin complexes (HIT)	Recent exposure to heparin	Platelet factor 4 antibody ELISA	Direct thrombin inhibitors

Granulocytes

Description

- Concentrate of white blood cells collected by apheresis
- Prepared from donors recently tested for viral markers
- Hematocrit: may be as high as 20%
- RBC crossmatching must be performed before transfusion
- Stem cell transplant patients need current forward and reverse typing (during engraftment period) to determine the "best" ABO match. Granulocytes cannot be washed.
- Stored at 20–24 °C and transfused ASAP; must be completed within 24 hours from collection

Indications

- Neutropenia ($< 0.5 \times 10^9$/L) and infection for $>$24–48 hours resistant to appropriate antibiotics or other modes of therapy, myeloid hypoplasia, and a reasonable chance for recovery of marrow function
- Neonatal sepsis with neutropenia
- Dose: 1×10^9 cells/kg

Summary of Blood Components

Table 16. Blood components

Product	*Volume*	*ABO/Rh Important?*	*Preparation Time*	*Storage After Issuing*	*Maximum Time to Transfuse*	*Expiration*	*Return to Blood Bank*
RBCs	250–330 mL (or aliquot)	Yes/yes	5–45 minutes; varies if antibodies present	BB-monitored refrigerator	4 hours	42 days from draw (AS)	30 minutes
FFP/FP24	200–350 mL	Yes/no	35 minutes	BB-monitored refrigerator	4 hours	24 hours from thaw	30 minutes
Cryo	10–15 mL	Yes/no	10–15 minutes	Room temperature	4 hours	6 hours from thaw	ASAP
Platelets	200–350 mL	Yes/yes	10 minutes	Room temperature	4 hours	5 days from draw	ASAP

Coagulation Factor Concentrates

Description

- Concentrates of coagulation factors prepared from human plasma or via recombinant technology
- Steps to increase safety of plasma (similar level of safety as recombinant products) (18):
  - Collected by apheresis of donors who test negative twice for viral markers prior to purification of factors (serologic and nucleic acid tests)
  - Manufacturing process involves viral inactivation steps: detergent-treatment or heat

Table 17. Coagulation factor concentrates and treatment indications

Disorder	*Product*	*Brand Names*	*Indication*	*Vial Label*
Hemophilia A	Recombinant factor VIII	Advate rAHF®, Helixate®, Kogenate®, Recombinate®, Refacto®	Previously untreated patients (PUPs)	Number of units of factor VIII
	High-purity factor VIII concentrate, plasma-derived	Hemofil-M®, Koate-HP®, Monoclate-P®, Monarc-M®	Patients previously exposed to plasma and/or with hepatitis B or C, or HIV infection	Number of units of factor VIII
	Intermediate purity factor VIII concentrate, plasma-derived	Alphanate®, Humate-P®	Mainly von Willebrand disease or same as high-purity plasma-derived	Number of units of von Willebrand factor and factor VIII
Hemophilia B	Recombinant factor IX	BeneFIX®	PUPs	Number of units of factor IX
	High-purity factor IX concentrate, plasma-derived	Alphanine SD®, Mononine®	Patients previously exposed to plasma and/or with hepatitis B or C, or HIV infection	Number of units of factor IX

Hemophilia A or B with inhibitor or acquired hemophilia*	Activated prothrombin complex concentrates	Factor VIII inhibitor bypass activity (FEIBA FH®)	Patients previously exposed to plasma and/or with hepatitis B or C, or HIV infection	Number of units
	Recombinant factor VII activated	NovoSeven®	PUPs	Vials of 1.2, 2.4, or 3.6 mg
Von Willebrand disease	Intermediate purity factor VIII concentrate, plasma-derived	Alphanate, Humate-P	Mainly von Willebrand disease or same as high-purity plasma-derived factor VIII	Number of units of von Willebrand factor and factor VIII
Other factor deficiencies (X and prothrombin)	Prothrombin complex concentrates	Profilnine, Bebulin VH®	Deficiencies of factor IX, X, or prothrombin	Number of factor IX units (variable amounts of X and II)

*Autoimmune disorder caused by sudden development of IgG anti-factor VIII. Usually in individuals >60 years of age, unless associated with pregnancy. *Dramatic* presentation with soft tissue or mucosal bleeding, mainly gastrointestinal and/or genitourinary.

Dose calculations for coagulation factors

- Dose depends on clinical indication for coagulation factor: prophylactic or therapeutic
- Based on normal factor levels: 50–150% activity for all factors or 0.5–1 unit/mL of plasma
- Minimum hemostatic level of every factor: 30% or 0.3 unit/mL of plasma
- Suggested peak factor levels for various indications:
    - Single joint bleeding: 30–50%
    - Intramuscular bleeding: 80–100%
    - Hematuria: 50%
    - Intracranial bleeding: 100%
    - Gastrointestinal bleeding: 50%
    - Minor surgery: 30% up to 3–4 days postoperative
    - Major surgery: 80% up to 4–5 days postoperative
- A peak factor level of 75% provides sustained minimum hemostatic level of 37.5% at trough, defined as lowest level prior to next dose
- How to calculate the dose of factor concentrates:
    1. Blood volume (BV) in mL = Weight (kg) × 70 mL/kg
    2. Plasma volume (PV) in mL = BV (mL) × (1 – hematocrit)
    3. Units of factor required for initial dose = (desired level in % activity – current level in % activity) × PV in mL
    4. Maintenance dose = 50% of initial dose
- Example of calculation:
  How much factor VIII should be given to a 50-year-old male, 83 kg, 40% hematocrit, with severe hemophilia A (factor VIII activity: <1%), no inhibitor, with hemarthrosis in the right knee, to raise his level to 75% or 0.75 units/mL?
    1. Blood volume (BV) in mL = 83 kg × 70 mL/kg = 5,810 mL
    2. Plasma volume (PV) in mL = 5,810 mL × (1 –.4) = 3,486 mL

3. Units of factor required for initial dose = (0.75 – 0) × 3,486 in mL = 2,600
4. Maintenance dose = 50% of initial dose = 1,300

- Issue factor vials that add up to the closest number of units possible.
- Give maintenance doses every 12 hours.
- Monitor factor VIII activity 15–30 minutes from initial dose (peak) and prior to next dose (trough) and make dose adjustments as needed.
- If patient developed inhibitor since last assay, peak level should be adequate but trough will be much lower than half of peak.
- If hematocrit changes due to bleeding or transfusion, recalculate plasma volume and dose accordingly.
- For hemophilia B patients:
  - Calculated dose should be doubled to account for factor loss in the extravascular space.
  - Half-life of factor IX is 24 hours; dose once a day
- For patients with von Willebrand disease:
  - Calculate dose of von Willebrand factor as for factor VIII.
  - Because VWF concentrates also have factor VIII, its level will increase further than expected based on the dose given because endogenous factor VIII will bind to infused von Willebrand factor.
- For patients with factor VIII (or IX) inhibitor:
  - FEIBA and NovoSeven are not dosed based on plasma volume, but in units/kg of body weight.
  - FEIBA guidelines:
    - Joint bleeding: 50 units/kg every 12 hours
    - Mucous membrane bleeding: 50 units/kg every 6 hours
    - Intramuscular bleeding: 100 units/kg every 12 hours
    - Total daily dose *must not exceed* 200 units/kg/24 hours as it causes risk of DIC.

- NovoSeven:
  - 90–120 μg/kg every 2–3 hours, depending on response
- No laboratory test needed to monitor response to FEIBA or NovoSeven (although PT and PTT will shorten, no correlation with clinical response, should not be used to evaluate effectiveness of treatment)
- Recent publication found FEIBA and NovoSeven equivalent to stop bleeding (19)

Blood Transfusion Therapy

Medical Decision to Transfuse

- Widespread need for formal training in transfusion medicine among all clinical specialties
- Most physicians learn from peers' experience, not from evidence
- Literature lacks definitive guidelines for proper use of blood products in many clinical conditions

Table 18. Literature review of red cell transfusion in critically ill patients: available evidence

TRICC trial: multicenter, randomized, controlled clinical trial of transfusion requirements in critical care (20)
Randomized, controlled trial conducted 1994–1997 • 418 patients assigned to restrictive strategy of transfusion when hemoglobin <7 g/dL to maintain at 7–9 g/dL • 420 patients assigned to liberal strategy of transfusion when hemoglobin <10 g/dL to maintain at 10–12 g/dL • 30-day mortality similar in the two groups (18.7% vs. 23.3%, p = 0.11) • 30-day mortality was significantly lower in the restrictive transfusion strategy among patients who were less acutely ill; APACHE II score <20 (8.7% vs. 16.1%, p = 0.03) • 30-day mortality lower in the restrictive group among patients <55 years of age (5.7% vs. 13%, p = 0.02)

(Continued)

Table 18. (Continued)

- Mortality among patients with cardiac disease did not differ at 30 days (20.5% vs. 22.9%, $p = 0.69$)
- Mortality rate during hospitalization was lower in the restrictive strategy group (22.2% vs. 28.1%, $p = 0.05$)
- Liberal group received a mean of 5.6 units of RBCs compared to 2.6 units in the restrictive group ($p < 0.01$)

ABC study: anemia and blood transfusion in critically ill patients (21)

Prospective observational study conducted in November 1999

- ICU stay and overall mortality rates were significantly higher in patients who received a transfusion (ICU rates: 18.5% vs. 10.1%, $p < 0.001$; overall rates: 29.0% vs. 14.9%, $p < 0.001$).
- For similar degrees of organ dysfunction, patients who had a transfusion had higher mortality rate.
- For matched patients in the propensity analysis, the 28-day mortality was 22.7% among patients with transfusions and 17.1% among those without ($p = 0.02$).

The CRIT study: anemia and blood transfusion in the critically ill; current clinical practice in the United States (22)

Prospective, observational cohort study conducted in 2000–2001

- Mean pretransfusion hemoglobin, 8.6 g/dL
- Number of RBC transfusions independently associated with longer ICU and hospital length of stay and increased mortality
- Patients who received transfusions had more total complications.
- A baseline hemoglobin level of <9 g/dL was a predictor of increased mortality and length of stay.

SOAP study: Is red blood cell transfusion associated with worse outcome? Results of the SOAP study (23)

Observational study from 2002

- Patients classified into those who received RBC transfusion during ICU stay and those who were not transfused

- Both ICU and hospital mortality rates were higher in transfused patients (23.0% vs. 16.3% and 29.9% vs. 22.5%, $p < 0.001$).
- Patients receiving ≥4 units had higher ICU and hospital mortality rates than those who received <4 units (28.6% vs. 18.0%, and 34.7% vs. 25.6%, $p < 0.01$).
- For patients matched according to a propensity score, ICU and hospital mortality rates were identical in transfused and non-transfused patients (22.7% vs. 22.1% and 29.1% vs. 29.0%, p = NS).
- Survival at 30 days was similar between the two matched groups.

The "transfusion dilemma"

- Optimal hemoglobin concentration varies considerably from patient to patient; hemoglobin concentration should not be guiding factor for the "transfusion trigger."
- Each patient must be individually assessed to determine his or her tolerance to anemia and need for transfusion.
- Clinical examination and background data, including current diagnosis and co-morbid conditions, must be evaluated.

Multiple factors to consider prior to transfusing

- Age
- Preexisting chronic disease, especially coronary, cerebrovascular, and respiratory
- Present diagnosis and severity
- Underlying cause of anemia
- Surrogate measures of tissue oxygenation: mixed venous oxygen saturation; blood lactate levels

Plasma products

- Much less data than for RBC transfusions (24)
- Associated with different risks: allergic reactions, TRALI, anaphylaxis (25)

- Coagulation screening tests, especially PT, commonly used to decide to transfuse plasma (26)
- Poor correlation between prolongations of PT and risk of bleeding

Platelets

Uncertain trigger; variable according to patient clinical situation (24,27)

Treatment of bleeding

Site or type of bleeding is good indicator to narrow therapeutic choices. Transfusion decision must take into account patient-specific situation, risks, benefits, and alternatives.

Transfusion Medicine Blood Specimen Requirements

Blood specimen quality

Safe blood transfusion and the accuracy of pretransfusion testing require absolute identification of the patient and a correctly labeled patient blood specimen. Specimens must be properly collected, labeled, stored, and transported. Procedures must be explicitly followed with "zero tolerance" for deviation. Shortcuts should never be taken, especially in emergency situations where errors are more likely to occur.

Transfusion request form

The transfusion request form accompanying the blood sample should contain sufficient information to positively identify the patient at the time of specimen collection, including two independent identifiers. Forms are unacceptable if they are incomplete, inaccurate, or illegible (8). The request form should contain the patient's full name, identification number, physician's name, number and type of component ordered, date of scheduled transfusion, and special instructions such as irradiation or leukocyte reduction. It is also useful to have the patient's age, date of birth, gender, diagnosis, and transfusion history.

Patient identification

If the patient is conscious and coherent, ask the patient to state and spell his/her full name and compare it to the transfusion request form and armband. If the patient is unable to identify him/herself, get confirmation of identity from a person familiar with the patient (28). An armband must be attached to the patient and used for identification, and the information must agree, item by item, with the information on the transfusion request. Discrepancies between the request form and the armband must be resolved before the specimen is collected. The information on the request form and the specimen label must be complete, accurate, and legible (8). For emergency situations, a temporary transfusion identification system must be used until the name and identity of the patient are established.

Specimen and labeling

Blood specimens for testing must have a label containing the date of collection and two independent identifiers (8), usually the patient's full name and medical record identification number. The completed label must be attached to the specimen before the phlebotomist leaves the patient. The label must be complete, accurate, and legible. There must be a mechanism to identify the phlebotomist. Either serum or plasma may be used for testing, depending on the institutional policy and the methodology employed.

Age of specimen

If the patient has been transfused or pregnant in the preceding three months, or if the history is unknown, the specimen must be obtained within three days of the transfusion (8).

Specimen identification in the transfusion service

The information on the blood specimen label and the transfusion request must be compared and confirmed to agree by the transfusion service before acceptance. Both the request form and the specimen label must be complete, accurate, and legible (8). If there is any discrepancy, the specimen cannot be accepted by the transfusion service and a new, properly labeled specimen must be collected. It is not acceptable to correct an incorrectly labeled specimen.

Pretransfusion Testing

Compatibility testing steps

- Determination of ABO and Rh type of donor (performed by collection facility and confirmed by transfusion service) and screen for unexpected antibodies (by the collection facility)
- Determination of ABO and Rh type of recipient
- Antibody screen to detect clinically significant antibodies in recipient
- Crossmatch to demonstrate compatibility between recipient and donor (for RBCs and granulocytes)
- Comparison of current test results with previous records of testing

ABO and Rh type

RBCs selected for transfusion are usually matched with the recipient's ABO and Rh type. In some instances, ABO-compatible units are given (see Table 24). The recipient's ABO type is determined by testing for antigens on the red cells with anti-A and anti-B reagents, and testing for the expected antibodies in the serum or plasma with A1 and B reagent red cells (8) (see Table 19).

Table 19. ABO types: antigens, antibodies, and frequencies

ABO Type	*Antigens on RBCs*	*Antibodies in Serum*	*Percent in United States*	
			Caucasian	*African-American*
O	None	anti-A and anti-B	45%	49%
A	A	anti-B	40%	27%
B	B	anti-A	11%	20%
AB	A and B	none	4%	4%

The Rh type is determined with anti-D reagent. All blood donors are tested for the D antigen and for weak D. If either test is positive, the unit is labeled "Rh Positive"; if both are negative, the unit is labeled "Rh Negative." It is not necessary to test for weak D in an apparent Rh-negative recipient. Rh-negative recipients should receive only Rh-negative RBCs, to avoid the risk of immunization to the D antigen. Rh-positive recipients can receive either Rh-positive or Rh-negative blood.

Rh Blood Group Terminology

- Genetics of Rh system
  - D locus: 2 alleles; *D* gene produces D antigen (Rh positive), *d* gene produces no antigen (Rh negative)
  - CE locus: 4 alleles; *Ce*, *cE*, *ce*, *CE* produce the corresponding antigens
- Fisher-Race (DCE or CDE) terminology
  - Five major antigens: D, C, E, c, e
  - Eight potential combinations or haplotypes based on presence of genes for these antigens (i.e., "DCe," "dce," etc.; see Table 20)
- Wiener (Rh-Hr) terminology
  - R: Rh positive, D antigen present
  - r: Rh negative; D antigen absent
  - Superscripts to R and r designate the CE antigens present:
    - 0 or no superscript: both c and e present
    - 1 or ′ (prime): C and e present

- 2 or ″ (double prime): E and c present
- z or y: both C and E present

Table 20. Rh-positive and -negative haplotypes

Rh-Positive Haplotypes			Rh-Negative Haplotypes		
R^0	Dce	Most common Rh-positive haplotype in African-Americans	r	dce	Most common Rh-negative haplotype
R^1	DCe	Most common Rh-positive haplotype in Caucasians	r′	dCe	Uncommon
R^2	DcE	Uncommon	r″	dcE	Uncommon
R^z	DCE	Very rare	r^y	dCE	Very rare

Donor units are not routinely typed for antigens other than ABO and D, since the immunogenicity of other blood group antigens is much lower (Table 21). For example, only 5% of K-negative recipients exposed to K-positive RBCs via transfusion or pregnancy will develop anti-K, compared to 50% of D-negative recipients exposed to D-positive RBCs. Antigen frequency also is a factor in the potential of developing alloantibodies. Although c antigen is the third most immunogenic antigen, 80% of the population is positive for c, and could not produce anti-c.

Table 21. Immunogenicity of blood group antigens (29)

Antigen (Blood Group System)	*Antigenic Sites per RBC*	*Percent Immunogenicity*
D (Rh)	10,000–35,000	50%
K (Kell)	6,000	5%
c (Rh)	37,000–85,000	2%
E (Rh)	450–25,600	1.7%
k (Kell)	3,500	1.5%

Antibody screen; indirect antiglobulin test

Purpose

Clinically significant antibodies are defined as those that can shorten survival of transfused red cells, or cause hemolytic disease of the newborn (see Table 22). Most patients lack significant antibodies, other than anti-A or anti-B. However, previous transfusion, pregnancy, or transplantation may immunize the patient to produce antibodies against other blood group antigens. The patient's serum or plasma must be tested for clinically significant unexpected antibodies using 2 or 3 group O reagent red cells (unpooled) that have been phenotyped for all the common blood group antigens (8).

Techniques

- Methods of testing must include incubation at 37 °C and an antiglobulin test.
- LISS: Low ionic strength additive solution. LISS potentiator reduces the ionic strength of the reaction medium and enhances the rate of binding of positively charged antibody molecules.
- PEG: Polyethylene glycol potentiator; promotes antibody uptake and enhances the strength of reaction
- Tube test: Serum and reagent red cells are placed in a tube, usually with a potentiator, and observed for agglutination and hemolysis in various phases. Tests must include incubation at 37 °C, washing to remove unbound protein, and addition of antiglobulin serum to detect antibody coating the red cells.
- Gel test: Serum and reagent red cells are added to an acrylamide gel column containing anti-IgG. After incubation, the tests are centrifuged to push the cells into the gel. Antibody-coated cells (positive test) are agglutinated by the anti-IgG and remain suspended within the column. If the reagent red cells are not coated with antibody (negative test), the red cells pass through the gel to form a pellet at the bottom of the column.

- Solid phase red cell adherence: Microtiter wells coated with red cell antigens are incubated with the serum. If antibody is present, it will attach to the antigen. After washing to remove unbound antibody, IgG-coated indicator cells are added and the wells are centrifuged. In a positive test, the indicator cells react with the antibody bound to the antigen, forming a diffuse pattern covering the well. In a negative test, the indicator cells do not react, and form a pellet at the bottom of the well.
- Enzyme tests: proteolytic enzymes such as ficin cleave negatively charged sialic acid from the red cell membrane and decrease the negative surface charge of the cell, promoting agglutination. Reactions with Rh and Kidd antibodies are enhanced. However, MNS and Duffy system antigens are destroyed by enzyme treatment of red cells, and antibodies to these antigens will not be detected.

Interpretation

If significant antibodies are detected, they should be identified by testing with a reagent red cell panel. Donor red cells should be phenotyped to select antigen-negative blood, and a complete antiglobulin crossmatch must be performed.

Antibody identification

Positive results in the antibody screen indicate the presence of an unexpected antibody in the recipient's serum. The antibody is identified by testing the serum or plasma with a panel of 8–20 reagent red cells that have been phenotyped for all the common blood group antigens. The antibody specificity is determined by comparing the pattern of reactions of the serum with the phenotypes of the red cells in the panel. For identity to be established, the serum should be reactive with all cells that have the antigen, and nonreactive with all cells that lack the antigen. Weak antibodies, multiple antibodies with overlapping patterns, autoantibodies,

Table 22. Clinical significance of blood group antibodies (30)

Clinically Significant Antibodies	*Possibly Significant When Reactive at 37 °C*	*Rarely Significant*
ABO	P_1	Le^b
Rh	Le^a	Xg^a
Kell	MN	Sd^a
Kidd	Lutheran	
Duffy		
Ss		

and antibodies to high-frequency antigens usually require additional specialized techniques for positive identification.

Once a significant antibody is identified, donor blood selected for transfusion must be phenotyped negative for the corresponding antigen.

Crossmatch

The crossmatch tests the recipient's plasma/serum with the donor's red cells. It is designed to detect antibodies in the patient's plasma against antigens on the donor red cells. Methods used must detect ABO incompatibility and clinically significant antibodies, including an antiglobulin test (8). However, if the recipient's antibody screen is negative and there is no history of previous blood group antibodies, the only required method is one that will demonstrate ABO incompatibility. Three types of serologic or electronic crossmatch procedures are described in Table 23.

Table 23. Comparison of crossmatch methods

Type of Crossmatch	*Procedure*	*Detects*	*Indication/ Requirements*
Immediate spin	Patient serum and donor red cells are mixed, centrifuged, and examined for agglutination or hemolysis	ABO incompatibility	When patient's antibody screen is negative, and there is no history of alloantibodies
Antiglobulin	Patient serum and donor red cells are incubated at 37 °C and an antiglobulin test is performed	Incompatibility due to ABO or other clinically significant antibodies	Must be performed if the patient's antibody screen is positive and/or the patient has a history of alloantibodies
Electronic	Computer system is used to verify ABO compatibility between donor and recipient	ABO incompatibility	When patient's antibody screen is negative, and there is no history of antibodies. Requires two separate determinations of ABO type, and extensive computer system validation

Type and screen

The patient's ABO and Rh type are determined, and an antibody screen is performed. If the screen is negative and there is no history of blood group antibodies, no further testing is done until blood is needed. At that time, ABO-compatible blood is selected and an immediate spin or electronic crossmatch is performed prior to release.

If the antibody screen is positive or if there is a history of antibodies, donor red cells are phenotyped and antigen-negative blood is selected. A complete antiglobulin crossmatch must be performed (8).

Transfusion of non-group-specific blood

In emergency or special circumstances it may be necessary to transfuse blood of a different type than that of the recipient. RBCs should not be transfused if they contain an antigen that the patient has an antibody against. Plasma should not be transfused in appreciable quantities if it contains an antibody against a recipient red cell antigen. Table 24 shows acceptable choices for transfusion of red cells or plasma.

Table 24. Optional ABO types for transfusion of red blood cells and plasma

Recipient Type	*RBCs No Foreign Antigen Infused*	*Plasma No Antibody Against Recipient RBCs Infused*
A	A or O	A or AB
B	B or O	B or AB
AB	AB, A, B, or O	AB
O	O	O, A, B, or AB

Additional Testing

Direct antiglobulin test (DAT)

The direct antiglobulin test detects *in vivo* coating of red cells with IgG antibody and/or complement. Polyspecific antiglobulin sera containing anti-IgG and anti-C3d is added to the patient's washed red cells. The test is typically positive in conditions shown in Table 25.

Table 25. Causes of positive DAT

Condition	*Cause*
Autoimmune hemolytic anemia	Autoantibody against patient's red cell antigen
Hemolytic disease of the fetus or newborn	Maternal antibody against infant's red cell antigen
Hemolytic transfusion reaction	Alloantibody against transfused donor red cell antigen
Drug-induced immune coating of RBCs	Antibody to drug or hapten

When the DAT is positive, monospecific anti-IgG and anti-complement reagents may be used to determine the type of protein bound to the red cells, as shown in Table 26.

Table 26. Interpretation of polyspecific and monospecific DAT

Polyspecific DAT	*Anti-IgG*	*Anti-Complement*	*Interpretation*
+	+	0	IgG present
+	0	+	Complement present
+	+	+	Both IgG and complement present

Elution

An elution is performed to remove IgG antibody from red cells that show a positive DAT. The antibody in the eluate, freed from red cells, can then be tested with reagent red cells to identify its specificity.

Autoadsorption

Most autoantibodies react not only with the patient's own red cells, but also with all other red cells tested. This makes it difficult to detect an underlying alloantibody. An autoadsorption is performed to remove the autoantibody from the serum so that it can be tested for the presence of a concurrent alloantibody. Autoadsorption is performed by incubating the patient's serum with autologous red cells under controlled conditions. Consequently, the autoantibody attaches to the patient's red cells, leaving the alloantibody free in the serum. After centrifugation and removal of the coated red cells, the adsorbed serum can be used for alloantibody detection and crossmatching. Several autoadsorptions may be necessary to remove a strongly reactive autoantibody. For patients with severe autoimmune hemolytic anemia, it is a challenge to obtain enough red cells to perform multiple adsorptions prior to transfusion.

If the patient has been transfused in the past 90 days, even small amounts of the transfused donor red cells in the patient's circulation could adsorb an alloantibody during autoadsorption procedures. Results should be interpreted with caution, recognizing that a negative result does not guarantee that no alloantibody is present.

Donor RBC phenotype

When a clinically significant antibody is detected in the patient's serum, donor units selected for transfusion must be negative for the corresponding antigen. Donor cells are tested with reagent antisera, using appropriate techniques and controls. Antigen frequencies and % donor blood compatible are shown in Table 27.

Table 27. Blood group systems and antigen frequencies

Blood Group System	*Antigen*	*Antigen Frequency, %**	*Donor Blood Compatible (Antigen-Negative), %*
Rh	D	85%	15%
	C	70%	30%
	E	30%	70%
	c	80%	20%
	e	98%	2%
Kell	K	9%	91%
	Kp^a	2%	98%
	Js^a	0.1% Caucasian 19.5% African-American	99.9% Caucasian 80% African-American
	k, Kp^b, Js^b	99.9%	0.1%
Duffy	Fy^a	66%*	34%
	Fy^b	85%*	15% 68% of African-Americans are Fy (a– b–)
Kidd	Jk^a	77%	23%
	Jk^b	72%	28%
MNS	M	78%	22%
	N	72%	28%
	S	55%	45%
	s	89%	11%
P	P_1	80%	20%
Lewis	Le^a	22%	78%
	Le^b	72%	28% 22% of African-Americans are Le (a– b–)
Lutheran	Lu^a	8%	92%
	Lu^b	99.9%	0.1%

*Caucasian frequencies in the United States, except where noted. Frequencies may differ in African-Americans, Hispanics, Asian-Americans, and other groups.

To determine the number of units to phenotype to find antigen-negative blood for a patient, divide the *number needed* by the *frequency of antigen-negative*, expressed as a decimal. For patients with multiple antibodies:

$$\frac{\text{Number of units needed}}{\%\ \text{antigen-negative} \times \%\ \text{antigen-negative}}$$

Antibody titer

IgG alloantibodies produced by pregnant women may destroy fetal red cells carrying the corresponding antigen, a condition known as hemolytic disease of the fetus and newborn (HDFN). These antibodies may be quantitated by antibody titration, in which serial dilutions of the maternal serum are tested with red cells positive for the antigen, by an antiglobulin technique using anti-IgG. The reciprocal of the highest serum dilution showing 1+ agglutination is the antibody titer. Titers of 16 or above, or a greater than fourfold increase in titers of two timed specimens, indicate that the fetus is at risk of HDFN. Because the antibody titer alone cannot predict the severity of HDFN, amniocentesis, ultrasound measurement of blood flow in the middle cerebral artery of the fetus, or percutaneous blood sampling should be performed to monitor anemia in the fetus. Intrauterine transfusion is indicated if the baby requires treatment before delivery.

Rh immune globulin

Rh immune globulin (RhIG) is concentrated IgG anti-D administered IM or IV to prevent immunization in an Rh-negative person exposed to Rh-positive blood.

Postpartum

RhIG is administered within 72 hours of delivery of an Rh-positive infant to an Rh-negative mother who has not been previously immunized to D. One dose of 300 µg prevents immunization to up to 30 mL of Rh-positive blood or 15 mL of red blood cells. Required testing is shown in Table 28.

Table 28. Rh immune globulin testing

Specimen	*Test*	*Criteria for RhIG*
Mother	Rh type If negative, test for weak D	Rh negative
Baby	Rh type If negative, test for weak D	Rh positive If infant's type is unknown, give RhIG
Postpartum maternal	Screen for FMH	If positive (≥10 mL FMH), perform KB to quantitate FMH. If KB is ≥30 mL, increase the dose of RhIG

Antenatal

RhIG may be given at 28 weeks' gestation to prevent immunization from occurring during pregnancy in Rh-negative women. RhIG will not harm the fetus, although some babies may have a weak positive DAT at birth. Since the half-life of IgG is 25 days, it is essential that women who have been given antenatal RhIG receive another full dose of RhIG after delivery. The antibody screen may be positive from antenatal RhIG, but this should be recognized as passive immunization, not active immunization.

First trimester

A microdose of 50 µg protects against immunization in Rh-negative women during first trimester fetal loss.

Fetal screen and Kleihauer-Betke

The fetal rosette test is a screening test that detects the presence of Rh-positive red cells in Rh-negative blood. The test is required on postpartum specimens from all Rh-negative women who have delivered an Rh-positive baby, to determine whether a large fetomaternal hemorrhage (FMH) has occurred. The rosette test is positive when a FMH of 10 mL or more has occurred during delivery.

In the rare instance where there has been an FMH greater than 30 mL, the dose of Rh immune globulin must be increased to protect the mother against immunization. A Kleihauer-Betke (KB) test is performed to quantitate the amount of FMH detected by a positive rosette test. While the rosette test detects Rh-positive red cells, the Kleihauer-Betke detects red cells carrying fetal hemoglobin (Hb F). The appropriate dose of Rh immune globulin (RhIG) for a large FMH is calculated as follows:

$$\text{Volume of FMH} = \%\ \text{fetal cells counted in KB} \times 50$$

$$\text{Number of vials of RhIG needed} = \frac{\text{Volume of FMH}}{30} + 1\ \text{vial}$$

The Kleihauer-Betke is occasionally performed on blood from pregnant women after trauma to identify whether there has been significant fetal bleeding. The test is not indicated for pregnancy less than 14–20 weeks, because the volume of the fetal blood is too small to detect an FMH.

Blood Administration Guidelines

Informed consent

Except for emergency situations, informed consent for transfusion must be obtained before the blood is administered. Policies must be developed by the facility in accordance with state and local laws. Informed consent policy should cover at least these areas (8):

- Description of the transfusion risks, benefits, and alternatives
- Opportunity for questions
- Right to accept or refuse transfusion

Physician's order

There must be a written physician order for transfusion. Before administering the blood, the transfusionist should check the physician's order and verify that the component to be transfused and the dose are correct (31).

Issuing blood for transfusion

Before the blood or component is issued, it must be inspected by qualified personnel. The information on the donor unit label, the attached compatibility label or tie tag, and the blood request information should be checked for accuracy and completeness. This includes the following (8,32):

- Recipient's name and second independent identifier
- Recipient's ABO and Rh type
- Donor unit or pool number
- Donor ABO and Rh type
- Interpretation of compatibility test, if performed
- Special component requirements:
  - Antigen-negative
  - Leukocyte reduced
  - CMV-negative
  - Irradiated
  - IgA-deficient donor
  - Uncrossmatched
- Date and time of issue
- Expiration date and time of donor unit
- Appearance of donor unit, comparing the unit and the attached segments:
  - Abnormal color—brown, black, or purple. Color of the blood in the bag should not be darker than the color of the blood in the segments
  - Clots
  - Hemolyzed or icteric plasma

- Leaks, air, or bubbles
- Visible clumps, in platelet products

The results of the inspection must be documented.

Return of unused blood; requirements for re-issue

Release blood may be returned to the blood bank or transfusion service for re-issue if it meets these requirements (8):

- The container has not been entered.
- The appropriate temperature of the component has not been exceeded. RBCs and thawed FFP must be maintained at 1–10 °C during transportation. As a general rule, refrigerated components can be outside the refrigerator for 30 minutes before 10 °C is exceeded. Platelets and cryoprecipitate are stored and transported at room temperature, 20–24 °C.
- At least one sealed segment remains attached to the returned unit.
- Return, inspection, and acceptability for re-issue are documented.

Recipient and donor unit identification at bedside

It is crucial that the recipient and donor be accurately identified before the blood is administered. Automated barcode scanners can be used to scan the patient's armband, the donor unit label, and the transfusionist's ID badge. The transfusionist must check all identifying information in the presence of the recipient, and sign the transfusion record verifying that the information is correct. Commonly, two individuals check the information together before transfusion. Information to be checked:

- Recipient identification: the two independent identifiers on the armband must match the two identifiers on the compatibility (transfusion) label or tie tag attached to the unit.
- Donor identification: the donor number or pool number on the bag label must match the number on the compatibility label.

- ABO and Rh: the ABO and Rh on the donor bag label must match the ABO and Rh of the donor on the compatibility label. The recipient's ABO and Rh type must be recorded on the compatibility label, although it may be different from the donor's ABO and Rh.
- Interpretation of the compatibility test must be recorded on the compatibility label.
- The expiration date of the donor unit must be checked on the donor bag label.

The compatibility label or tie tag must remain attached to the unit throughout the transfusion (8).

Other preinfusion checks

The transfusionist should:

- Verify that there is a physician order for the transfusion and that informed consent has been obtained.
- Check for any special processing requests such as leukoreduction or irradiation.
- Observe the appearance of the unit and check the bag for leaks.

Patient monitoring

The patient's baseline vital signs (temperature, pulse, respiration, and blood pressure) should be obtained before transfusion, and checked again after the transfusion (8). Many institutions check the vital signs after the first 15 minutes of transfusion and every hour thereafter, until one hour following transfusion. The blood should be started slowly and the patient observed carefully for the first 15 minutes of transfusion, when most serious reactions are manifest. If there are any signs and symptoms of a reaction at any time, the transfusion should be stopped and a transfusion reaction investigation initiated.

Rate and time of infusion

Blood administration should begin within 30 minutes of issuing the blood from the transfusion service. For routine transfusions, the blood should be infused slowly during the first 15 minutes, <5 mL/minute. Blood can then be administered as rapidly as the patient can tolerate, but most RBC transfusions are given within 1–2 hours. Transfusion must be completed within 4 hours (8).

Needle and catheter size

Using 18- to 20-gauge needles and catheters is recommended for routine transfusion of adults (32). Pediatric patients or patients with limited venous access may be transfused using 23- to 25-gauge needles or vascular catheters, although the flow rate will be slower.

Filters

Blood and components must be infused though a filter designed to remove clots and cellular debris. Types of filters:

- Standard blood transfusion sets: 170–260 micron pore size filter in blood administration set removes clots and other debris. Most standard sets can be used to filter 2–4 units of red cells, however, the filter should be used for no longer than 4 hours (33).
- Microaggregate filters: 20–40 micron pore size. These filters are designed to trap microaggregates of platelets, leukocytes, and fibrin formed in RBCs stored longer than 5 days (33).
- Leukocyte reduction filters: selectively reduce leukocytes in RBCs and platelet components to $<5\times10^6$. Red cell leukocyte filters and platelet leukocyte filters cannot be used interchangeably. Leukocyte reduction or microaggregate filters must not be used for transfusion of granulocytes (33).

Infusion devices, blood warmers

Controlled infusion devices and infusion pumps may be used to regulate the flow of blood, if tested and used as specifically recommended by the manufacturer. Blood warmers are sometimes used to prevent hypothermia in exchange transfusions, massive transfusions, and patients with cold agglutinin disease. To prevent hemolysis, blood warmers must be tested and monitored to ensure that temperatures do not exceed manufacturers' specifications.

IV solutions and medications

An IV solution of 0.9% USP normal saline is acceptable for infusing with blood, priming filters, or diluting RBCs units. Addition of normal saline to RBCs may be desirable to reduce viscosity and improve the flow rate. Medications and drugs should never be added to blood or components unless they have been approved by the FDA for this use, or there is documented evidence of the safety of this practice (8). Even then, it would be preferable to infuse medication through a separate IV line to monitor the dosage in the event of infusion problems.

Lactated Ringer's solution should not be used with blood transfusion, because it contains calcium, which may cause clotting (28,33). A solution of 5% dextrose in water (D5W) is contraindicated because it may cause clumping and hemolysis of red cells.

Outpatient transfusions

If direct medical observation or patient monitoring is not available for an appropriate time after the transfusion, the patient or caregiver should be given written instructions for signs and symptoms of delayed adverse reactions. Include the telephone number and name of the healthcare provider in case problems or questions arise.

Transfusion documentation in medical record

- Transfusion order
- Component name
- Donor unit or pool identification number
- Date and time of transfusion
- Pre- and posttransfusion vital signs
- Amount transfused
- Identification of the transfusionist
- Adverse transfusion events, if applicable

Urgent Requirement for Blood (8)

Request

In urgent situations, blood may be issued before standard compatibility or infectious disease tests are completed. Transfusion service records must contain a signed statement from the physician indicating that the clinical situation is sufficiently urgent to warrant release of products before completion of testing.

Laboratory testing and selection of blood

- If there is not time to determine the recipient's ABO type, group O RBCs should be issued.
- If possible, Rh-negative RBCs should be selected, especially for women of childbearing age whose Rh type is unknown.
- If the recipient's ABO type has been determined by testing a current specimen, type-specific or type-compatible RBCs should be issued.
- Compatibility testing using a properly labeled specimen and standard techniques should be completed as soon as possible. The physician should be notified of any problems or incompatibility.

Unit label

A conspicuous label or tie tag must be attached to the donor unit indicating that compatibility and/or infectious disease testing is incomplete.

Massive Transfusion

Description

Massive transfusion is defined as transfusion of an amount of blood equal to or greater than the patient's blood volume (10 units in an adult) within a 24-hour period (Table 29). Exchange transfusion of an infant is a massive transfusion

Table 29. Parameters associated with increasing severity of hemorrhagic shock (34)

Parameter	*Class I*	*Class II*	*Class III*	*Class IV*
% of blood volume lost	<15%	15–30%	31–40%	>40%
Pulse (bpm)	<100	>100	>120	>140
Blood pressure (mmHg)	Normal	Normal	Decreased	Decreased
Respiratory rate (breaths/min)	14–20	20–30	30–40	>35
Fluid replacement	Crystalloid	Crystalloid	Crystalloid and blood	Crystalloid and blood

Laboratory testing

After a massive transfusion, both pretransfusion blood specimens and current blood specimens have limited usefulness in testing. Pretransfusion testing may be abbreviated to confirm only ABO compatibility in subsequent transfusions (35). Written laboratory procedures/policies should be established for compatibility testing in instances of massive transfusion.

Complications

- Stored RBCs do not contain platelets or labile coagulation proteins. Transfusion of platelets and FFP or FP24 may be indicated to correct dilutional coagulopathies (33).
- Hypothermia
- Citrate toxicity leading to hypocalcemia
- Hypomagnesemia
- Hyperkalemia

Intrauterine Transfusion

Selection of RBCs

- Type O Rh negative
- Negative for antigen corresponding to mother's antibody
- CMV seronegative or leukocyte reduced
- Hemoglobin S negative
- Less than 7 days old, for optimal 2,3-DPG level and viability

Pretransfusion testing

- Negative for antigen reactive with mother's antibody
- Crossmatch compatible with maternal serum or plasma
- Gamma irradiated to prevent GVHD

Transfusion techniques

- Intraperitoneal
- Intravascular (umbilical vein)

Exchange Transfusion of Infants

Selection of RBCs

- Baby's ABO type if compatible with mother; otherwise, type O
- Rh negative if mother has anti-D; otherwise, baby's Rh type

- Negative for antigen reactive with mother's antibody
- CMV seronegative or leukocyte reduced
- Hemoglobin S negative
- Less than 7 days old, for optimal 2,3-DPG level and viability

Pretransfusion testing

- Negative for antigen reactive with mother's antibody
- Crossmatch compatible with maternal serum or plasma
- Gamma irradiated to prevent GVHD

Transfusion techniques

- Continuous infusion
- Intermittent withdrawal and infusion using syringe

Transfusion in Neonates (Less Than 4 Months)

Guidelines

The neonatal period is from birth to four months of age. Hospitalized infants undergoing laboratory testing often need transfusion to replace blood lost by repeated sampling. Alloimmunization during this period is very unlikely, due to the infant's immature immune system. Therefore, only limited pretransfusion testing need be performed.

Transfusion of 5–15 mL/kg of RBCs should raise the infant's hemoglobin approximately 3 g/dL (36).

Initial pretransfusion testing

ABO type

- Test infant's red cells with anti-A and anti-B reagents.
- Reverse typing is not indicated.
- For A, B, or AB neonates whose mother is ABO incompatible, if other than group O RBCs will be transfused:

  - The neonate's serum or plasma must be tested for passively acquired anti-A or anti-B, using reagent A_1 or B cells, or the donor's cells, by the antiglobulin method.
  - If anti-A or anti-B is detected, units lacking the corresponding antigen should be selected for transfusion.

Rh type

- Test the infant's red cells with anti-D reagent.
- The test for weak D is not indicated.

Antibody screen

- Perform on the serum or plasma of either the infant or the mother
- If the antibody screen is negative, no crossmatch is necessary for the initial or repeat transfusions.
- If the antibody screen is positive, units selected for transfusion should be either:
  - Negative for the corresponding antigen, or
  - Compatible by the antiglobulin crossmatch

Crossmatch

- Not required if antibody screen is negative (see Antibody Screen above)

Repeat transfusion testing

- Repeat ABO, Rh, antibody screen, and crossmatch are not required for neonates if the initial antibody screen is negative.
- If the original antibody screen is positive, either antigen-negative donor units or antiglobulin-crossmatch-compatible donor units should be given for as long as the antibody is detectable.

Additional considerations for neonatal transfusion

- HGB S negative
- CMV negative: safe for infants weighing less than 1200 g
- Donor RBCs <7 days old:
  - Several studies document the safety of RBCs stored up to 42 days using AS-1 anticoagulant (see Table 9), which contains both adenine and mannitol as preservatives (37).
  - Extracellular potassium (K^+) rises with extended storage. In CPDA-1, K^+ rises to 78 mmol/L by day 35. In AS, K^+ rises to 45–50 mmol/L by day 42 (38).
  - Irradiation may double extracellular K^+, thus RBCs may need to be washed depending on the child's K^+ level.
  - No significant change in K^+ concentration after small volume (10–20 mL/kg) transfusions given over 2–3 hours
  - K^+ problematic in massive transfusion: cardiopulmonary bypass, ECMO, or exchange transfusion. Use units <1 week old, or washed if fresh not available
- Several small-volume aliquots from the same donor will limit donor exposure and risks; "dedicated unit" protocol.
- Guidelines and indications for RBC transfusion (39):
  - HGB <13 g/dL (HCT <40%) with severe cardiopulmonary disease
  - HGB <10 g/dL (HCT <30%) with moderate cardiopulmonary disease or surgery
  - HGB <8 g/dL (HCT <24%) with symptomatic anemia
  - Bleeding or phlebotomy exceeding 25% of red cell volume

Platelet transfusion in neonates

- Usual dose is 5–10 mL/kg of platelets
- Like RBC, may require irradiation

- Triggers for platelet transfusion in neonates (39):
  - Platelet count <100,000/μL with bleeding or clinically unstable, including intraventricular hemorrhage
  - Platelet count <50,000/μL prior to an invasive procedure
  - Platelet count <20,000/μL even without bleeding and clinically stable

Pediatric Transfusion (Older Than 4 Months)

Selection of RBCs

- ABO type-specific or ABO compatible
- Rh-negative recipients should receive only Rh-negative RBCs. Rh-positive recipients can receive either Rh-positive or Rh-negative blood.

Pretransfusion testing

- Compatibility testing and antibody detection requirements are the same as for adult patients.

Transfusion considerations

- Differences in blood volumes and ability to tolerate blood loss
- Differences in normal hemoglobin and hematocrit for age level (see Table 30)

Table 30. Hemoglobin and hematocrit reference ranges for children (40)

	1–3 Years	*4–7 Years*	*8–13 Years*
HGB, g/dL	9.6–15.6	10.2–15.2	12.0–15.0
HCT, %	34–48	36–46	35–49

Adverse Effects of Blood Transfusion

Patient management

- Monitor patient carefully during transfusion.
- Stop the transfusion at first sign or symptom of an adverse reaction.
- Re-check the identification of the patient and donor unit; verify that the unit is correct.
- Notify the patient's physician and the transfusion service.
- Maintain IV fluids and urinary output; monitor and maintain vital signs.
- Collect posttransfusion blood and urine samples.
- Complete the transfusion investigation request, documenting patient symptoms, vital signs, and the amount of blood transfused.
- Send to the transfusion service:
    - Postreaction blood and urine samples from the patient
    - Transfusion reaction investigation request
    - Blood bag with attached administration set and IV solutions

Laboratory investigation

- Perform clerical check of records and labels to verify correct identification of patient and donor.
- Centrifuge postreaction blood sample and examine serum/plasma for hemolysis. If noted, compare with pre-reaction specimen.
- Perform direct antiglobulin test (DAT). If positive, compare with prereaction specimen DAT.
- Repeat the ABO type on the posttransfusion blood sample.
- If there is evidence of a hemolytic transfusion reaction, additional testing should be performed, as needed:
    - Repeat ABO type of the donor unit and pretransfusion patient sample
    - Repeat antibody screen on the pre- and posttransfusion sample
    - Repeat crossmatch with the pre- and posttransfusion samples

- Perform antibody identification and/or elution studies if unexpected antibody is detected by the antibody screen or DAT.
- Phenotype the donor unit for the corresponding antigen.
- Test for evidence of red cell hemolysis, such as haptoglobin, plasma hemoglobin, bilirubin at 5–12 hours, hematocrit, LDH.
- Perform coagulation tests for DIC: PT, APTT, fibrinogen, platelet count.

- If there are signs of a bacterial reaction, perform Gram stain and culture of the donor unit.
- If there are indications of TRALI, rule out other potential adverse causes such as acute HTR and sepsis (41).
  - Postreaction complete blood count (CBC) may show leukopenia in TRALI cases (42,43).
- Notify the patient's physician immediately if the investigation suggests an acute hemolytic reaction, bacterial contamination, TRALI, or other serious transfusion reaction.

Table 31 shows causes, symptoms, laboratory findings, and methods of prevention of immediate adverse reactions to blood transfusion. Delayed transfusion complications and risks of transfusion-transmitted viral infections are shown in Tables 32 and 33.

Treatment

- Treat shock and support cardiac and respiratory function.
- Maintain renal output.
- Treat DIC, if present.
- For bacterial contamination/sepsis: broad spectrum antibiotics and resuscitative therapy
- For TRALI: supplemental oxygen, IV fluids to maintain blood pressure, possible intubation
- For febrile nonhemolytic reaction: antipyretics
- For circulatory overload: diuresis, phlebotomy

Table 31. Immediate adverse reactions

Type	*Cause*	*Symptoms*	*Laboratory Findings*	*Prevention*
Hemolytic (HTR)	Antibody to donor red cell antigen, causing intravascular or extravascular hemolysis; activation of complement and/or coagulation systems, generation of inflammatory cytokines	Fever and chills Dyspnea Hypotension Shock Red or brown urine Chest and lower back pain Nausea and vomiting DIC Renal ischemia and failure	DAT mixed field positive Antibody screen positive or negative (ABO incompatibility) Plasma hemolyzed Falling hematocrit Haptoglobin decreased LDH increased Bilirubin increased	Proper identification Adherence to policy and procedures for specimen collection, testing, and administration
Febrile nonhemolytic (FNHTR)	Cytokines accumulated during storage of donor blood Patient antibodies to donor WBCs or platelets	Temperature rise of more than 1 °C or 2 °F, within 2 hours of transfusion, not associated with another cause Chills, rigors	Transfusion reaction investigation: Negative for HTR	Prestorage leukocyte reduced blood products Premedication with acetaminophen

Allergic	Reaction to plasma protein or other soluble component	Urticaria, itching, rash Wheezing	Transfusion reaction investigation: Negative for HTR	Premedication with antihistamine Washed RBCs
Anaphylactic	Anti-IgA or another antibody Severe allergic reaction occurs immediately after transfusion of small amount of donor blood	No fever Hypotension, shock Respiratory distress, dyspnea Sweating, flushing, nausea, vomiting, abdominal cramps Substernal pain	Transfusion reaction investigation: Negative for HTR IgA deficiency with anti-IgA	Antihistamines, epinephrine, steroids Washed or IgA-negative blood products (see *Transfusion Therapy in Specific Diseases—IgA Deficiency*)
Bacterial	Transfusion of contaminated blood (more likely with platelets; see *Pheresis Platelets, BDS testing*)	High fever Chills Hypotension, Shock Vomiting, diarrhea DIC	Transfusion reaction investigation: Negative for HTR Gram stain and culture positive	Aseptic blood collection Proper storage BDS testing Inspection of unit for abnormal color and clots Administer blood product within 4 hours of issue or pooling

(Continued)

Table 31. (Continued)

Type	*Cause*	*Symptoms*	*Laboratory Findings*	*Prevention*
Transfusion-related acute lung injury (TRALI)	Donor-derived granulocyte-specific or HLA class I antibodies to recipient antigens, mediate WBC agglutination and inflammatory response causing plasma leakage from damaged capillaries into the lungs	Onset within 6 hours of transfusion Dyspnea, hypotension Pulmonary edema Pulmonary artery pressure <18 mm Hg Ratio PaO_2/FIO_2 <300 mm Hg, or O_2 sat <90% Fever	Transfusion reaction investigation: Negative for HTR Chest radiograph: bilateral pulmonary infiltrates	Deferral of donors previously implicated in TRALI Transfusion of plasma from male donors or donors who have not been previously transfused or pregnant
Transfusion related circulatory overload (TACO)	Rapid infusion Excess volume transfused	Nonproductive cough Cyanosis Dyspnea, rales Hypertension, rapid pulse Congestive heart failure	Transfusion reaction investigation: Negative for HTR	Slow infusion of blood products and IV fluids

Table 32. Delayed complications of transfusion

Type	*Cause*	*Symptoms*	*Laboratory Findings*	*Treatment or Prevention*
Delayed hemolytic	Recipient previously immunized Antibody no longer detectable Blood with corresponding antigen is transfused Anamnestic response; extravascular hemolysis occurs 2–14 days after transfusion	Fever Decreasing hematocrit Anemia Mild jaundice	DAT mixed field pos Antibody screen may be pos or neg Falling hematocrit Haptoglobin decreased LDH, bilirubin may be elevated	Check of previous records before transfusion
Post-transfusion purpura (PTP)	Platelet alloantibody (usually anti-HPA-1) in recipient destroys autologous platelets after transfusion	Severe thrombocytopenia 8–10 days after transfusion	Transfusion reaction investigation: Negative Platelet antibody screen and identification	High dose IVIg Plasmapheresis

(Continued)

Table 32. (Continued)

Type	*Cause*	*Symptoms*	*Laboratory Findings*	*Treatment or Prevention*
Transfusion-associated graft-vs.-host disease (TA-GVHD)	Donor T-lymphocytes engraft in recipient and mount immune response against recipient tissue, including hematopoietic blood cells	Fever Rash Severe diarrhea Hepatitis Infectious or hemorrhagic complications from pancytopenia	Pancytopenia	Prevention: Irradiation of all components for at-risk patients, including immuno-compromised patients, related donors, and HLA-selected products (See *Irradiated Blood Products*)
Disease transmission	Viruses: HAV, HCV, HBV, HDV, HIV, HTLV-I/II, CMV, EBV, B19 parvovirus, WNV Parasites: T. cruzi, Babesia, malaria Prions: CJD, vCJD	Hepatitis: fever, anorexia, nausea, vomiting, malaise HIV/AIDS: fever malaise, arthralgias, infections, lymphadenopathy	Clinical symptoms and positive laboratory tests for infectious agent	Accurate and thorough donor medical history Disease testing of donor blood Leukocyte reduction

Alloimmunization to red cell or HLA antigens	Immune response to foreign antigens	Positive red cell antibody screen or Positive platelet antibody screen	For some diseases involving chronic transfusion, such as sickle cell anemia, phenotype-matched blood may prevent alloimmunization

Table 33. Risks of transfusion-transmitted viral infections (44,45)

Infection	*Approximate Risk of Disease Transmission Per Unit Transfused*
HIV-1	1: 2,000,000
HCV	1: 2,000,000
HBV	1: 205,000
HTLV	1: 3,000,000

Transfusion Therapy in Specific Diseases

Autoimmune hemolytic anemia (46)

- Two main types of autoimmune hemolytic anemia (AIHA):
  - Warm: IgG anti-RBC antibodies; optimally bind at core body temperature (37 °C)
    - Most common form of AIHA, about 70%
  - Cold: IgM anti-RBC antibodies; react more strongly at 4 °C
    - Cold AIHA is also known as cold agglutinin disease (CAD)
  - Both can be primary or secondary to other conditions or drugs
- Laboratory features and type of hemolysis:
  - Positive direct antiglobulin test (DAT) or direct Coombs test; sine qua non criterion
    - Warm type DAT positive for IgG only, or IgG plus C3, or C3 only (less often); extravascular hemolysis predominantly
    - CAD: DAT positive for C3 (IgM activates complement quite efficiently); intravascular hemolysis
    - The stronger the DAT, the higher the association with hemolysis.
  - Positive antibody screen; serum reactive with full panel, including auto control

- Primary objective of pretransfusion testing is to detect any underlying alloantibody that may be masked by the presence of autoantibody
- Anemia with microspherocytes (warm AIHA) or with red cell agglutination (CAD)

Table 34. Assays used in the evaluation of patients with AIHA

Test	*Comments*
DAT: polyspecific and monospecific	Assesses for IgG and/or C3 on the cell membrane. Small number of cases of AIHA may have negative result (below sensitivity of the assay)
Elution	Removes the IgG autoantibody from the red cell so its specificity can be evaluated. If DAT is only weakly positive for IgG, eluate may be negative
Antibody screen; if positive, reagent red cell panel	Checks for auto and/or alloantibody(ies) in patient's serum. May be negative if all autoantibody bound to RBCs (usually accompanying weak positive DAT)
Autoadsorption	Serum is adsorbed with patient red cells. Removes autoantibody from serum to allow detection of residual alloantibody(ies) (if present). If recent transfusion (previous 90 days), adsorption may also remove alloantibody(ies)
Alloadsorption	Serum is adsorbed with either red cells of the same phenotype as the patient, or with aliquots of R^1R^1, R^2R^2, and rr red cells, in an attempt to remove the autoantibody and detect underlying alloantibody. Used in patients with recent transfusion or severe anemia (blood volume for autoadsorption not obtainable)

(Continued)

Table 34. (Continued)

Test	*Comments*
Thermal amplitude	Determines the range of reactivity of cold agglutinins. Antibody is clinically significant if reactive at ≥30 °C
Crossmatch	Likely to be incompatible with straight serum but compatible with adsorbed serum. Prewarmed crossmatch can be used in CAD to exclude alloantibodies

Transfusion support in AIHA

- Decision to transfuse must be made on a case-by-case basis: not based on degree of anemia
- Life-threatening hemolysis: harmful to withdraw transfusion due to incompatible crossmatches
- Communication between transfusion service and clinical team crucial to understand risks, benefits and alternatives of transfusion (release form may be used to document discussion)
- Transfused cells will have shortened survival to the same extent as patient's own cells
- Incompatible units with nonadsorbed (straight) serum have risk of alloantibody-mediated hemolysis (unless patient never transfused or pregnant previously)
- Blood warmer may be used for patients with CAD

Sickle cell anemia (SCA) (47,48)

- Incidence: 1 in 500 of African-Americans; sickle cell trait: 1 in 12 African-Americans
- Severe chronic hemolysis due to poorly deformable RBCs containing 100% of hemoglobin S
  - Hemoglobin S: $\beta^{6Glu \rightarrow Val}$: valine is substituted for glutamine at the sixth position of the β-chain

- When deoxygenated, HGB S forms insoluble linear crystals that distort RBCs into sickle shape, occluding vessels and causing hemolysis.
- Transfusion in SCA: prophylactic or therapeutic
- Prophylactic RBC transfusions decrease hemoglobin S concentration to prevent complications such as stroke, splenic sequestration, and intractable pain, and prior to angiography.
- Therapeutic transfusions:
  - Acute: aplastic crisis, acute chest syndrome, acute splenic sequestration, sepsis, acute papillary necrosis, stroke, priapism, intractable pain crisis
  - Chronic: pregnancy, hematuria, chronic renal or cardiac failure, preoperative period, skin ulcer
    - Transfusion during pregnancy may be warranted in patients with other risk factors such as multiple gestation or history of previous fetal loss.
    - Preoperative RBC transfusion indicated when general anesthesia expected. Simple or exchange transfusion depending on time and availability. Desired HGB S concentration: 30–40% and total hemoglobin: 11–13 g/dL. Hypoxemia, dehydration, acidosis, and hypothermia must be avoided to prevent sickling during surgery.
- Selection of blood donors:
  - Negative for sickle cell trait: units must be screened prior to transfusion
  - Leukoreduction decreases alloimmunization against HLA
  - Full red blood cell phenotype indicated prior to initiating transfusions
    - In some centers, units are routinely matched for C, E, and Kell, in addition to ABO and D.
  - Overall risk of alloimmunization: 20–30%; most common antibodies to Rh, Kell, and Kidd antigens

    - Difference in antigen frequencies and immunogenicity of various RBC antigens account for risk of alloimmunization
  - Some patients form multiple antibodies: very difficult to find compatible units
    - Most donors in the United States are Caucasians

IgA deficiency (49)

- IgA deficiency with concomitant lack of secretory IgA: most common primary immunodeficiency in the Western world
- IgA level <7 mg/dL in males or females >4 years with:
  - Normal serum IgG and IgM
  - No other explanation for hypogammaglobulinemia
- Severe IgA deficiency: selectively undetectable IgA concentration of <0.05 mg/dL
  - American Red Cross Rare Donor Program (ARDP) uses this definition to classify blood donors as IgA deficient
- Incidence of IgA deficiency varies with population examined, analytical sensitivity of method used to screen individuals, and cut-off value used to classify individuals as IgA deficient
  - Available methods to measure IgA in serum and their lower detectable limits:
    - Nephelometry: 6–7 mg/dL
    - Passive hemagglutination inhibition (PHAI): 0.05 mg/dL
    - ELISA: 0.005 mg/dL
- Frequency of anti-IgA in IgA-deficient individuals can range from 11.5% to 46.8%
- Unclear which stimuli lead to the production of anti-IgA antibodies. Some cases associated with a history of exposure to IgA antigen from a variety of sources

- Serum anti-IgA antibodies sine qua non for the diagnosis of anaphylactic transfusion reactions in IgA-deficient patients
  - Preformed antibodies to transfused IgA may be class-specific (anti-IgA), subclass-specific (Anti-IgA_1 or -IgA_2), or allotype-specific [Anti-$IgA_{2m(1)}$ or anti-$IgA_{2m(2)}$]
  - Most severe anaphylactic transfusion reactions usually associated with class-specific antibodies in severely IgA-deficient patients
  - Subclass and allotype-specific antibodies, also called antibodies of "limited specificity," associated with less severe transfusion reactions, frequently seen in patients with low or, in some instances, normal levels of IgA
- IgA anaphylactic transfusion reactions are rare:
  - Estimated occurrence rate of 1:20,000 to 1:100,000 transfusions
  - Prevalence of major anaphylactic transfusion reactions in the United States population approximately 2.4%
  - No documented cases of mortality due to anti-IgA-associated anaphylactic transfusion reactions
  - Frequency of detecting anti-IgA (1:1,200) exceeds observed frequency of anaphylactic transfusion reactions, suggesting that anti-IgA in a patient's serum is not good predictor of the risk for an anaphylactic transfusion reaction
- Prior to transfusion:
  - Screen with nephelometry.
  - If IgA <7 mg/dL, test with more sensitive assay.
  - If IgA level <0.05 mg/dL, test for antibodies.
  - If anti-IgA present, use autologous transfusions, washed RBC units, or any products from IgA-deficient donors.
  - In an emergency, with no time to wait on more sensitive assay:
    - No history of anaphylactic reaction, low risk of anaphylaxis (1:20,000–1:100,000 transfusions)

- With history of anaphylactic reaction, use only autologous transfusions, washed RBC units, or any products from IgA-deficient donors.
- Platelets and plasma must be from IgA-deficient donors.
- Beware that IV immunoglobulin, Rh immune globulin, factor VIII concentrates, and albumin may contain sufficient amounts of IgA to trigger reactions.

Neonatal alloimmune thrombocytopenia (NAIT)

- Caused by maternal alloantibodies to fetal platelet antigens
- Most common antigen implicated: HPA-1
- High frequency antigen in general population
- May occur in the first pregnancy when fetus carries the antigen from father
- Subsequent children likely to be affected
- Fetal platelet count may be monitored during third trimester
  - Obstetricians may request HPA-1 negative platelets for intrauterine transfusion
    - Unit must be O negative or positive, CMV-negative and irradiated
    - In the absence of suitable donor, collect mother's platelets by apheresis or from whole blood donation—antibody present will not affect survival of transfused cells
    - Some hospitals concentrate platelets from 100 mL of the unit immediately prior to transfusion
- Delivery of affected children often by cesarean section to avoid bleeding complications
- Immediate postnatal platelet count checked
- Compatible platelet units ready to be transfused if needed
- Close coordination with obstetrical team is necessary to provide product when needed and avoid wasting unique platelet product

Bone marrow and hematopoietic stem cell transplantation

- Allogeneic transplant of ABO mismatched pairs: transfused products must be compatible with patient's circulating cells and antibodies.
- Know patient (recipient)'s historical blood type, donor's type, and date of transplant.
- Repeat type and screen every 3 days to verify forward and reverse results.
- Check DAT if antigen and antibody(ies) (anti-A and/or anti-B) are present concurrently.
- Decide on the best option for transfusion, shown in Table 35.

Table 35. Transfusion options for recipients of ABO-mismatched transplant

			FFP and Platelets			
Recipient	*Donor*	*RBCs*	*1st*	*2nd*	*3rd*	*4th**
O	A	O	A	AB	B	O
O	B	O	B	AB	A	O
O	AB	O	AB	A	B	O
A	O	O	A	AB	B	O
B	O	O	B	AB	A	O
AB	O	O	AB	A	B	O
A	B	O	AB	A	B	O
B	A	O	AB	B	A	O
A	AB	A	AB	A	B	O
B	AB	B	AB	B	A	O
AB	A	A	AB	A	B	O
AB	B	B	AB	B	A	O

*Issue low titer (<50) for 2nd–4th choices of platelets

Therapeutic Apheresis

- Apheresis means "to take away" (Greek)
- Two main types of therapeutic apheresis:
  - Blood component exchanges: plasmapheresis, red cell exchange
  - Cell depletions: leukepheresis, plateletpheresis
- Other modalities:
  - Photopheresis or extracorporeal photochemotherapy (ECP)
  - Selective removal by adsorption, such as low-density lipoprotein (LDL) apheresis
- Two types of technology to perform therapeutic apheresis:
  1. Centrifugation: Cobe Spectra (Gambro BCT), CS3000 (Fenwal), AS104 (Fresenius), MCS + LN9000 (Haemonetics)
     - Most commonly used in North America
     - Separation of blood components based on density: red cells >granulocytes >monocytes >lymphocytes >platelets > plasma
     - Continuous or discontinuous flow: former more efficient
     - Whole blood collected though inlet, mixed with anticoagulant (commonly acid-citrate-dextrose-formula A), taken into chamber to be separated into various component layers
     - Outlet tubing can remove any blood element, depending on type of procedure; remaining components are returned to patient mixed with replacement plasma, 5% albumin or red cells (in plasma or red cell exchanges, respectively).
  2. Membrane filtration: Plasmaflo (Asahi) and Prisma TPE (Gambro BCT)
     - Only for plasma exchange
     - Uses membranes permeable to high-molecular-weight proteins but not cells

- Typical set-up: blood pump, anticoagulant pump (usually heparin), replacement fluid pump, and effluent pump
- No need for centrifugation and citrate; allows for faster procedures

Indications should be based on three types of evidence (50)

- Known pathogenesis
  - Secure understanding of disease process should suggest a clear rationale for the therapeutic apheresis modality such as conditions known to be "caused" by an excess of a circulating blood cell or by a circulating antibody
  - Example: Leukostasis in acute leukemia
- Proven effect
  - Clear evidence that abnormality that makes apheresis plausible can be corrected by therapeutic apheresis
  - Candidate pathogenic molecules large enough to be mostly present intravascularly
    - Only substances consistently removed are large macromolecules with relative long half-lives and slow resynthesis, like IgG or low density lipoproteins
  - Example: Hyperviscosity syndrome: excess immunoglobulin, usually IgM, causes increased plasma volume with subsequent end-organ damage
- Improved patient outcomes
  - Strong evidence that therapeutic apheresis leads to clinically significant benefit, not just statistically significant results
  - Prior to submitting patient to therapeutic apheresis, consider the following compared to other available therapies:

- Effectiveness
- Risk/benefit ratio
- Cost/benefit ratio
- Inconvenience/benefit ratio

  - Example: Goodpasture's syndrome or anti-glomerular membrane antibody syndrome

- All three criteria are surprisingly difficult to fulfill:
  - Rigorous clinical trials had disappointing results despite strong rationale in some diseases.
  - In other cases, marginally significant evidence of clinical benefit may be considered suspicious because of lack of strong rationale.
  - Examples: Hyperviscosity syndrome or leukostasis syndromes, Goodpasture's disease, cryoglobulinemia, and Guillain-Barré syndrome
- American Society for Apheresis (ASFA) categories (see www.apheresis.org):

  I: Apheresis is an *established therapy* as shown by controlled studies.

  II: Apheresis is an *acceptable therapy* but is supportive to other first-line therapies.

  III: *No controlled studies* are available to support the efficacy of Apheresis.

  IV: Apheresis is of *no benefit*.

  Previous classification published in 2000; revised in 2007 (51).

Table 36. Category I indications for different modalities of therapeutic apheresis

Apheresis Modality	*Diseases*
Plasma exchange	Thrombotic thrombocytopenic purpura (TTP); hyperviscosity syndrome; antiglomerular basement membrane antibody disease (Goodpasture's syndrome); myasthenia gravis; acute inflammatory demyelinating polyradiculoneuropathy (Guillain-Barré); chronic inflammatory demyelinating polyradiculoneuropathy (CIDP); multiple sclerosis (relapsing, progressive); PANDAS*; and Sydenham's chorea
RBC exchange	Severe and acute thrombotic event in sickle cell disease
Cytapheresis	Hyperleukocytosis
Photopheresis	Cutaneous T cell lymphoma, prophylaxis of rejection postheart transplant
Selective adsorption	Familiar hypercholesterolemia

*PANDAS, pediatric autoimmune neuropsychiatric disorders associated with streptococcal infections.

Therapeutic plasma exchange (TPE) (52)

By far, most commonly used type of therapeutic apheresis

Volume of plasma

- Usually 1–1.5 plasma volumes (PV)—essential to calculate for each patient
- Larger volume exchanges less efficient and increase risk of side effects
    - 1.0 PV exchange leaves 35% of original plasma
    - 1.5 PV exchange leaves 20% of original plasma
    - 2.0 PV exchange leaves 12% of original plasma

Table 37. Efficiency of removal of specific plasma proteins by a one-plasma volume removal (53)

Constituent	*Decrease, %*	*Recovery in 48 Hours, %*
Clotting factors	25–40%	80–100%
Fibrinogen	63%	65%
Immunoglobulins	63%	45%
Paraproteins	25–30%	Variable
Liver enzymes	55–60%	100%
Bilirubin	45%	100%
C3	63%	60–100%

- Percent decrease affected by distribution between intra- and extravascular spaces, and percent recovery depends on balance of synthesis, catabolism, and re-equilibration between compartments
- Volume exchanged aimed at maximum efficiency with minimal side effects such as dilutional coagulopathy and bleeding when using 5% albumin as replacement for plasma

Schedule of treatments

- Rarely enough to perform one exchange
- Based on ability of protein of interest such as IgG to re-equilibrate into the vascular space; typically takes 48 hours
    - Example:
        - IgG anti-acetylcholine receptor in myasthenic crisis at 10 g/L (assume only 45% intravascular)
        - 1 PV leads to 3.7 g/L
        - After re-equilibration at 48 hours: 7.2 g/L
        - If the goal of therapy is 70–85% reduction of intravascular level: 4 times 1 PV exchanges required; in practice, 5–6 exchanges plus immunosuppression needed for clinical benefit

- IgM more efficiently removed due to predominant intravascular distribution; requires fewer procedures
- Daily TPE is the gold standard for TTP (54):
  - Complex pathogenesis: TPE likely to remove IgG anti-von Willebrand cleaving protease (ADAMTS-13) and ultra-large multimers of von Willebrand factor (55,56)
  - Continued until platelet count reaches approximately 150,000/μL and no evidence of hemolysis; stable hemoglobin and normal LDH level
  - Perform few more TPEs every 48–72 hours (tapering period)
  - If response to initial treatment poor, may need intensification of PV exchanged (1.5 vs. 1.0) or initiation of immunosuppressive agents

Replacement fluid

- For most indications, 5% albumin:
  - Must use plasma for TTP (57); replenishes VWF-cleaving protease (ADAMTS-13)
  - Add plasma for high risk of bleeding due to coagulopathy (i.e., liver cirrhosis), active bleeding in Goodpasture syndrome, or TPE immediately pre- or postoperatively
  - Alternative to 5% albumin not widely used: hydroxethyl starches
  - If starting from 25% albumin, must dilute with saline to avoid hemolysis

Table 38. Advantages and disadvantages of albumin versus plasma

Replacement Fluid	*Advantages*	*Disadvantages*
5% albumin	Iso-oncotic, no viral risk, no contaminating "inflammatory mediators"	Higher cost than plasma, no coagulation factors or immunoglobulins
Plasma: FFP, FP24, CPP	Maintains normal levels of immunoglobulins, complement, coagulation factors	Viral transmission and ABO incompatibility risks, allergic reactions, high citrate load; large amount of sodium citrate: 14% by volume

- When using albumin, fibrinogen monitoring prior to each TPE avoids risk of bleeding:
  - If fibrinogen below 150 mg/dL consider addition of plasma at the end (final 1/3 PV)
  - Patients with liver impairment, including passive congestion, recover fibrinogen slower than normal

Potential complications of TPE (58)

- Therapeutic apheresis procedures are quite safe with mostly mild complications.
- Overall incidence of mostly reversible adverse effects 4.75%
- Types of side effects:
  - Physiologic: coagulopathy, decrease in cell counts or immunoglobulins, metabolic alkalosis
  - Unexpected: respiratory distress, arrhythmia
  - Mild: citrate toxicity, catheter site pain
  - Severe: anaphylactic transfusion reaction

- Possible complications of TPE:
  - Fluid imbalance: hypotension
  - Citrate effects: see below
  - Vasovagal effects: pallor or diaphoresis, nausea/vomiting, syncope and/or seizure
  - Venipuncture: severe pain, nerve damage, palpable hematoma
  - Central access: infection, thrombosis, pneumothorax or hemothorax, other hemorrhage, arterial puncture
  - Other severe events: chills/rigors, arrhythmia (non-citrate-related), transfusion reaction, anaphylaxis, viral transmission from plasma
  - Severe cardiorespiratory events: respiratory distress, circulatory collapse, cardiac arrest, death
  - Malfunctions: hemolysis, air embolus, clot/leak, unable to return blood
- How to predict which patients will have an adverse event:
  - Patient-specific factors:
    - Anxiety level, age, gender, diagnosis, concurrent problems, medications, size, blood and plasma volume, blood pressure, cardiac, hepatic and renal function, type of venous access
  - Procedure-associated factors:
    - Albumin versus plasma, rate of exchange, anticoagulant infusion rate, frequency of treatments
- How to avoid untoward events:
  - *Talk to patient:* Explain procedure, answer questions, anticipate anxiety, reassure patient of safety
  - Limit number of people in room: close family and apheresis personnel
  - Maintain a calm atmosphere: speak softly and show confidence on ability to perform treatment
  - If unexpected event happens, explain exactly what is going on
  - Reassure patient you know how to handle unexpected event and complete procedure
  - *Stay calm and show compassion*

- Symptoms of hypocalcemia and citrate toxicity:
  - Mild:
    - Numbness or tingling around the mouth and face
    - Sneezing
    - Chewing on the lips
  - Moderate:
    - Paresthesia progressing to hands, feet, and/or chest
    - Chills despite use of blood warmer
    - Nausea and vomiting, abdominal cramping
    - Vibrating sensation
    - Lightheadedness and mild hypotension
    - Restlessness
  - Severe:
    - Muscle cramps, severe abdominal cramping
    - Tremors
    - Bladder and/or bowel incontinence
    - Fear of impending doom
    - Loss of consciousness
    - Blurred or double vision
    - Severe hypotension; systolic BP <90 mm Hg, sudden onset
    - Cardiac: arrythmia, bradycardia, prolonged QT interval, premature ventricular contractions (PVCs)
    - Neuromuscular irritability such as *Chvostek's sign:* tap the mandibular joint and the face will grimace; or *Trousseau's sign:* inflate the blood pressure cuff and the hand muscles will cramp; or seizures
- Unusual reaction during TPE with albumin:
  - Albumin may contain FXII fragments serving as prekallikrein activator, along with low levels of bradykinin and kallikrein.

- Patients on angiotensin-converting enzyme (ACE) inhibitors will accumulate bradykinin: hypotension and bradicardia.
  - Avoid use of ACE-inhibitors in patients undergoing TPE
  - If patient already on ACE-inhibitor, recommend stopping drug 24 hours to several days before procedure (depending on drug half-life)

Red blood cell exchange (RCE)

Indications

- Serious complications in sickle cell disease patients (47):
  - Acute chest syndrome
  - Primary or secondary prevention of stroke
  - Retinal infarction
  - Persistent priapism not responding to conservative treatment
  - Repeated intractable pain crisis resistant to standard management
  - Pregnancy and prior to surgical procedures requiring prolonged general anesthesia—sometimes indicated
- As a mode of chronic transfusion to remove old RBCs while transfusing new RBC:
  - STOP clinical trial documented the ability to predict which children were at risk for stroke, allowing therapeutic intervention (chronic transfusion) *before* this devastating complication (59)
- Isovolemic RBC transfusion for overwhelming hemolytic parasitic infection of red cells:
  - Malaria
  - Babesiosis

Goals of RCE

- Rapid removal of sickle cells
- Maintenance of both HCT and HGB S concentration $<30\%$

Prior to procedure

- Know patient's height, weight, current HCT, percentage of HGB S
- Apheresis instrument calculates volume of RBCs needed for RCE
- Requirements for units used for RCE:
    - Negative for HGB S; screened with solubility test
    - Fresh, <7 days old
        - Contain at least half of initial 2,3 DPG concentration; better oxygen-carrying capacity
        - Have longer survival in circulation
    - Leukoreduced
        - To avoid febrile transfusion reaction during RCE
        - To decrease HLA alloimmunization
    - May be phenotype-matched with patient: Rh and Kell antigens matched resulted in small rate of sensitization (2%) versus 20% in non-matched transfusions (60)

Photopheresis

- Immunotherapy that combines leukapheresis with photochemotherapy
- Approved by Food and Drug Administration for cutaneous T cell lymphoma (CTCL)
- Also used in recipients of solid organs, mainly heart and lungs, with the following goals:
    - Prevent rejection
    - Treat acute and chronic rejection
    - Decrease risk of rejection in high-risk hypersensitized patients
    - Reduce intimal hyperplasia postcardiac transplant
    - Reduce drug immunosuppression

Procedure

- Whole blood collected into instrument (UVAR, Therakos)
- Centrifuged and WBC collected in satellite bag; RBCs and plasma returned to patient
- 3–6 cycles of buffy coat collection depending on patient blood volume and hematocrit
- WBCs exposed to injectable 8-methoxypsoralen
- Irradiated with ultraviolet A light; 1–2 J/cm^2 inside instrument
- Photoactivation time depends on treatment volume, hematocrit of buffy coat, and intensity of light bulb
- Methoxypsoralen-treated cells returned to patient

General mechanism of action of photopheresis in CTCL (61)

- Lymphocytes exposed to psoralen and ultraviolet-A irradiation undergo apoptosis
- Circulating monocytes undertake massive transformation into immature dendritic cells (DCs)
- Newly formed DCs phagocytize and internalize apoptotic cells, process their antigens, and increase the synthesis of class I and II major histocompatibility complex (MHC) molecules which are presented to CD4+ T helper cells
- DCs mature through a variety of mechanisms, including CD40 ligation
- Mature DCs fully loaded with pathogenic T cell peptides migrate to secondary lymphoid organs, stimulate naive CD8+ T cells
- CD8 cells induce response against pathogenic clones that express relevant peptides

General mechanism of action of photopheresis in management of rejection of solid organs (62)

- Similar to CTCL, except induction of stimulation of the immune system to destroy T cells causing allograft rejection ("transimmunization") instead of the malignant clones
- Induction of antigen-specific immunotolerance via expansion of regulatory T cells (T regs)

Alternatives for Patients Who Refuse Transfusion

- See Rogers DM, Crookston KP. The approach to the patient who refuses blood transfusion. Transfusion 2006;46:1471–7 (63)
- Similar principles applicable to patients with multiple antibodies to common antigens
- Develop a rapport with the patient and understand his/her reasons to refuse transfusion.
- Document discussion with patient.
- Maintain strict confidentiality and respect for patient's position.
- Make contingency plans for the future.
- Limit blood draws to a minimum and use pediatric tubes for essential laboratory tests.
- For specific questions regarding Jehovah's Witnesses, contact experienced physicians at 718-560-4300 or e-mail his@jw.org.
  - Products never accepted: any allogeneic blood component and autologous units
  - Generally accepted options:
    - Preoperative and intraoperative blood conservation measures
    - Volume expanders: saline, lactated Ringer's, hydroxyethyl starches
    - Antifibrinolytics

    - Hematopoietic growth factors
    - Albumin-free coagulation factors
    - Topical hemostatic agents
- Consult the Society for the Advancement of Blood Management *(http://www.sabm.org)* and the Network for Advancement of Transfusion Alternatives *(http://www.nataonline.com).*
- Blood substitutes not available for clinical use; under research protocol

References

1. Dzik WH. Emily Cooley Lecture 2002: Transfusion safety in the hospital. Transfusion 2003;43:1190–9.
2. Brown MR, Fritsma MG, Marques MB. Transfusion safety: what has been done; what is still needed? Med Lab Obs 2005;37:20–6.
3. McClelland DB, Phillips P. Errors in blood transfusion in Britain: survey in hospital haematology departments. BMJ 1994;308:1205–6.
4. Sazama K. Reports of 355 transfusion-associated deaths: 1976 through 1985. Transfusion 1990:30:583–90.
5. Linden JV, Wagner K, Voytovich AE, Sheehan J. Transfusion errors in New York state: an analysis of 10 years' experience. Transfusion 2000; 40:1207–13.
6. Linden JV, Kaplan HS. Transfusion errors: causes and effects. Transfus Med Rev 1994;8:169–83.
7. Code of federal regulations. Title 42 CFR 640.3. Washington, DC: U.S. Government Printing Office, 2006 (revised annually).
8. Silva MA, ed. Standards for blood banks and transfusion services, 24th ed. Bethesda, MD: AABB, 2006.
9. AABB & Food and Drug Administration. Blood donor history questionnaire Version 1.2, Feb 2007. http://www.aabb.org/Content/Donate_Blood/Donor_History_Questionnaires/AABB_Blood_Donor_History_Questionnaire/dhq.htm (Accessed March 2007).
10. American Red Cross. Blood donation eligibility guidelines. http://www.redcross.org/services/biomed/0,1082,0_557_,00.htmL #inf (Accessed March 2007).
11. AABB. Medication deferral list, June 2005. http://www.aabb.org/Documents/Donate_Blood/Donor_History_Questionnaire/udhqmeddefv1–2.pdf (Accessed February 2007).
12. AABB. The 2005 nationwide blood collection and utilization survey report. http://www.aabb.org/Content/About_Blood/FAQ/bloodfaq.htm (Accessed March 2007).
13. O'Neill EM, Rowley J, Hansson-Wicher M, McCarter S, Ragno G, Valeri CR. Effect of 24-hour whole-blood storage on plasma clotting factors. Transfusion 1999;39:488–91.

14. Cardigan R, Lawrie AS, Mackie IJ, Williamson LM. The quality of fresh frozen plasma produced from whole blood stored at 4 °C overnight. Transfusion 2005;45:1342–48.
15. Downes KA, Wilson E, Yomtovian R, Sarode R. Serial measurement of clotting factors in thawed plasma stored for five days. Transfusion 2001;41:570.
16. Cid J, Lozano M, Fernandez-Aviles F, Carreras E, Pereira A, Mazzara R, Ordinas A. Anti-D alloimmunization after D-mismatched allogeneic hematopoietic stem cell transplantation in patients with hematologic diseases. Transfusion 2006;46:169–73.
17. Cid J, Ortin X, Elies E, Castella D, Panades M, MartinVega C. Absence of anti-D alloimmunization in hematologic patients after D-incompatible platelet transfusions. Transfusion 2002;42:173–6.
18. Centers for Disease Control and Prevention (CDC). Blood safety monitoring among persons with bleeding disorders—United States, May 1998–June 2002. MMWR 2003;51:1152–4.
19. Astermark J, Donfield SM, DiMichele DM, Gringeri A, Gilbert SA, Waters J, et al. A randomized comparison of bypassing agents in hemophilia complicated by an inhibitor: the FEIBA NovoSeven Comparative (FENOC) Study. Blood 2007;109:546–51.
20. Hebert PC, Wells G, Blajchman MA, Marshall J, Martin C, Pagliarello G, et al. A multicenter, randomized, controlled clinical trial of transfusion requirements in critical care. N Engl J Med 1999;340:409–17.
21. Vincent JL, Baron JF, Reinhart K, Gattinoni L, Thijs L, Webb A, et al. Anemia and blood transfusion in critically ill patients. JAMA 2002;288: 1499–507.
22. Corwin HL, Gettinger A, Pearl RG, Fink MP, Levy MM, Abraham E, et al. The CRIT Study: Anemia and blood transfusion in the critically ill—current clinical practice in the United States. Crit Care Med 2004; 32:39–52.
23. Vincent et al. Is red blood cell transfusion associated with worse outcome? Results of the SOAP study. Chest 2003;124:125S.
24. Segal JB, Dzik WH. Transfusion medicine/hemostasis clinical trials network. Paucity of studies to support that abnormal coagulation test

results predict bleeding in the setting of invasive procedures: an evidence-based review. Transfusion 2005;45:1413–25.
25. Gajic O, Dzik WH, Toy P. Fresh frozen plasma and platelet transfusion for nonbleeding patients in the intensive care unit: benefit or harm? Crit Care Med 2006;34(5 Suppl):S170–3.
26. Abdel–Wahab OI, Healy B, Dzik WH. Effect of fresh-frozen plasma transfusion on prothrombin time and bleeding in patients with mild coagulation abnormalities. Transfusion 2006;46:1279–85.
27. Stanworth SJ, Hyde C, Heddle N, Rebulla P, Brunskill S, Murphy MF. Prophylactic platelet transfusion for haemorrhage after chemotherapy and stem cell transplantation. Cochrane Database Syst Rev 2004: CD004269.
28. AABB. Identification and safety. In: Primer of blood administration. http://www.aabb.org (Accessed February 2007).
29. Scott MD, Murad KL. Cellular camouflage: fooling the immune system with polymers. Curr Pharm Des 1998;4:423–38.
30. Garraty G. Mechanisms of immune red cell destruction and red cell compatibility testing. Hum Pathol 1983;14:209.
31. Brecher ME, ed. Administration of blood and components. In: Technical Manual, 15th ed. Bethesda, MD: AABB Press, 2005:521–32.
32. AABB. Blood administration practices. In: Primer of blood administration. www.aabb.org (Accessed February 2007).
33. Brecher ME, ed. Blood transfusion practice. In: Technical Manual, 15th ed. Bethesda, MD: AABB Press, 2005:483–514.
34. Davis KA, Gamelli RL. Transfusion therapy in the care of trauma and burn patients. In: Simon TL, Dzik WH, Snyder EL, et al., eds. Rossi's principles of transfusion medicine, 3rd ed. Philadelphia: Lippincott Williams & Wilkins, 2002:632–43.
35. Brecher ME, ed. Pretransfusion testing. In: Technical Manual, 15th ed. Bethesda, MD: AABB Press, 2005:407–20.
36. Brecher ME, ed. Neonatal and pediatric transfusion practice. In: Technical Manual, 15th ed. Bethesda, MD: AABB Press, 2005:557–77.
37. Strauss RG, Burmeister LF, Johnson K, James T, Miller J, Cordle DG, et al. AS-1 red cells for neonatal transfusions: a randomized trial assessing donor exposure and safety. Transfusion 1996;36:873–8.

38. Brecher ME, ed. Collection, preparation, storage, and distribution of components from whole blood donations. In: Technical Manual, 15th ed. Bethesda, MD: AABB Press, 2005:175–202.
39. Strauss RG. Neonatal transfusion. In: Anderson KC, Ness PM, eds. Scientific Basis of Transfusion Medicine: Implications for Clinical Practice, 2nd ed. St. Louis, MO: W.B. Saunders Company, 2000.
40. Rodak BF, Fritsma GA, Doig K. Hematology Clinical Principles and Application, 3rd ed. Philadelphia: Saunders Elsevier, 2007.
41. Kleinman S, Caulfield T, Chan P, Davenport R, McFarland J, McPhedran S, et al. Toward an understanding of transfusion-related acute lung injury: statement of a consensus panel. Transfusion 2004; 44:1774–89.
42. Nakagawa M, Toy P. Acute and transient decrease in neutrophil count in transfusion-related acute lung injury: cases at one hospital. Transfusion 2004;44:1689–94.
43. Marques MB, Tuncer HH, Divers SG, Baker AC, Harrison DK. Acute transient leukopenia as a sign of TRALI. Am J Hematol 2005;80:90–1.
44. Busch MP, Glynn SA, Stramer SL, Strong DM, Caglioti S, Wright DJ, et al. A new strategy for estimating risks of transfusion-transmitted viral infections based on rates of detection of recently infected donors. Transfusion 2005;45:254–64.
45. Dodd RY, Notari IV, Stramer SL. Current prevalence and incidence of infectious disease markers and estimated window-period risk in the American Red Cross donor population. Transfusion 2002;42:975–9.
46. Reardon JE, Marques MB. Laboratory evaluation and transfusion support of patients with autoimmune hemolytic anemia. Am J Clin Pathol 2006;125(Suppl 1):S71–7.
47. Sarode R, Altuntas F. Blood bank issues associated with red cell exchanges in sickle cell disease. J Clin Apher 2006;21:271–3.
48. Sharon BI, Honig GR. Management of congenital hemolytic anemias. In: Simon TL, Dzik WH, Snyder EL, et al., eds. Rossi's Principles of Transfusion Medicine, 3rd ed. Philadelphia: Lippincott Williams & Wilkins, 2002:463–82.
49. Lum G, Szuflad P, D'Amarino M. A patient with a low IgA level requiring transfusion during CABG surgery. Lab Medicine 2005;36:353–6.

50. McLeod B. An approach to evidence-based therapeutic apheresis. J Clin Apher 2002;17:124–32.
51. Szczepiorkowski ZM, Bandarenko N, Kim HC, Linenberger ML, Marques MB, Sarode, R, et al. Guidelines on the use of therapeutic apheresis in clinical practice—evidence-based approach from the Apheresis Applications Committee of the American Society for Apheresis. J Clin Apher 2007; 22:106–75.
52. Brecher ME. Plasma exchange: why we do what we do. J Clin Apher 2002;17:207–211.
53. Weinstein R. Basic principles of therapeutic blood exchange. In: McLeod BC, Price TH, Weinstein R, eds. Apheresis: Principles and Practice, 2nd ed. Bethesda: AABB Press, 2003:295–320.
54. Rock G, Shumak KH, Buskard NA, Blanchette VS, Kelton JG, Nair RC, Spasoff RA. Comparison of plasma exchange with plasma infusion in the treatment of thrombotic thrombocytopenic purpura. N Engl J Med 1991;325:393–7.
55. Furlan M, Robles R, Galbusera M, Remuzzi G, Kyrle PA, Brenner B, et al. von Willebrand factor-cleaving protease in thrombotic thrombocytopenic purpura and the hemolytic-uremic syndrome. N Engl J Med 1998;339:1578–84.
56. Tsai H-M, Lian E C-Y. Antibodies to von Willebrand factor-cleaving protease in acute thrombotic thrombocytopenic purpura. N Engl J Med 1998;339:1585–94.
57. Rock GA, Shumak KH, Buskard NA, Blanchette VS, Kelton JG, Nair RC, et al. Comparison of plasma exchange with plasma infusion in the treatment of TTP. N Engl J Med 1991;325:393–7.
58. McLeod BC, Price TH, Owen H, Ciavarella D, Sniecinski I, Randels MJ, Smith JW. Frequency of immediate adverse effects associated with apheresis donation. Transfusion 1998;38:938–43.
59. Lee MT, Piomelli S, Granger S, Miller ST, Harkness S, Brambilla DJ, et al. Stroke prevention trial in sickle cell enemia (STOP): extended follow-up and final results. Blood 2006;108:847–52.
60. Pugh TM, Johnson ST, Curnes JS, Weber KM. Reducing red cell alloimmunization in patients with sickle cell disease: a nine-year follow-up. Transfusion 2004:44(Suppl):135A.

61. Edelson RL. Transimmunization: the science catches up to the clinical success. Transfus Apher Sci 2002;26:177–80.
62. Lamioni A, Parisi F, Isacchi G, Giorda E, Di Cesare S, Landolfo A, et al. The immunological effects of extracorporeal photopheresis unraveled: induction of tolerogenic dendritic cells in vitro and regulatory T cells in vivo. Transplantation 2005;79:846–50.
63. Rogers DM, Crookston KP. The approach to the patient who refuses blood transfusion. Transfusion 2006;46:1471–7.

INDEX

A

B

C

D

F

G

H

I

N

O

P

R

S

T

U

V

W

Y